Hot Stone
and
Gem Massage

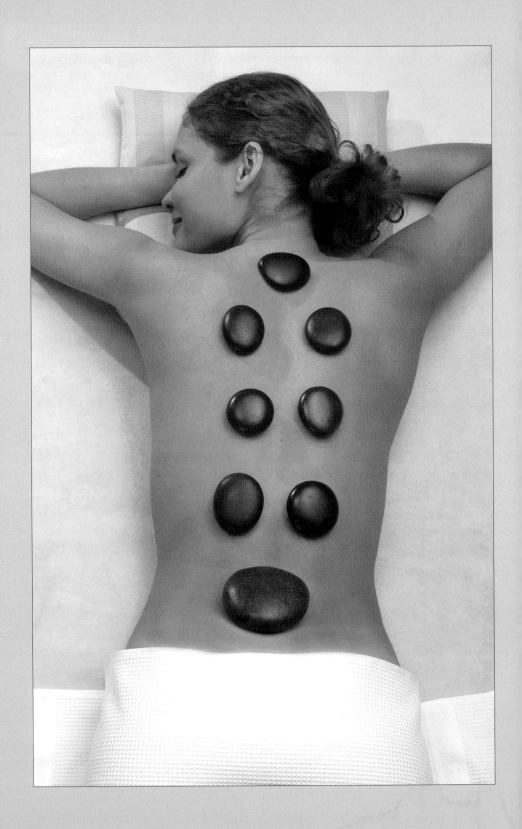

Hot
Stone
and
Gem
Massage

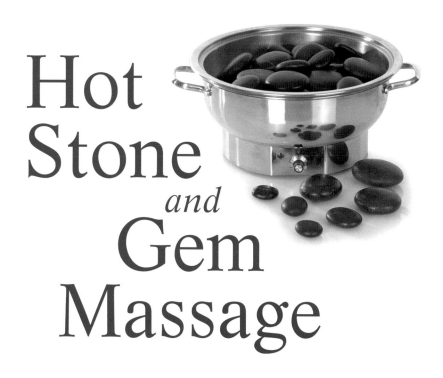

Dagmar Fleck and Liane Jochum

Translated from the German
by Nikolas Win Myint

Health
MASSAGE

Healing Arts Press
Rochester, Vermont

nlni
7/09

Healing Arts Press
One Park Street
Rochester, Vermont 05767
www.HealingArtsPress.com

Healing Arts Press is a division of Inner Traditions International

Originally published in German under the title *Hot Stones: Massagen mit heißen Steinen* by
Neue Erde
First U.S. edition published in 2008 by Healing Arts Press

*Note to the reader: This book is intended as an informational guide. The remedies, approaches,
and techniques described herein are meant to supplement, and not to be a substitute for, professional medical care or treatment. They should not be used to treat a serious ailment without
prior consultation with a qualified health care professional.*

Library of Congress Cataloging-in-Publication Data
Fleck, Dagmar.
  [Massagen mit heissen Steinen. English]
  Hot stone and gem massage / Dagmar Fleck and Liane Jochum ; translated from the
German by Nikolas Win Myint.
      p. cm.
  Originally published in German under the title: Hot Stones: Massagen mit heissen Steinen.
Neue Erde, c2006.
  Includes index.
  Summary: "A fully illustrated guide to the ancient Hawaiian art of massage with hot
stones"—Provided by publisher.
  ISBN 978-1-59477-246-7 (pbk.)
  1. Hydrostone therapy. 2. Massage. I. Jochum, Liane. II. Title.
  RM723.H93F5413 2008
  615.8'22—dc22
                                                                        2008025667

Printed and bound in India by Replika Press Pvt. Ltd.

10   9   8   7   6   5   4   3   2   1

Text design and layout by Virginia Scott Bowman
This book was typeset in Garamond Premiere Pro with Life and Stone Sans as display
typefaces
Photographs by Ines Blersch unless otherwise noted on page 140.

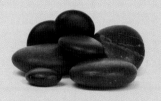

Contents

4 Hot Stone and Gem Massage

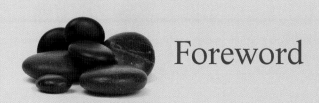

Foreword

Massage is something that you can begin to learn but you can never finish. The experience continues to deepen and become more intensive. Massage is one of the most subtle arts, and is not simply a question of technical skill. It is a question of love.

Osho

TOUCH IS ONE OF THE MOST POWERFUL METHODS of healing. To some extent this is due to the effects of the energy being exchanged, but probably more important is the bridge that touch creates between two living beings.

Society today is characterized by the term *individualization*. Individualization refers to a process in which traditional family and social circles have become so loose that people are increasingly left to rely on only themselves. In such a world of isolation and separateness, touch is a wonderful opportunity to create connection. Being touched by another can lead to physical, emotional, and mental changes in a person. The effect of one body on another is so powerful that for centuries it was denied, ritualized, or repressed.

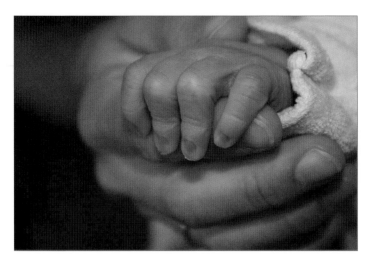

The power of touch

Different cultures have different customs for touching one another. Among the British and French, ritual touching through shaking hands or a quick kiss or near-kiss on one or both cheeks is common. The Japanese, on the other hand, avoid physical contact in public, preferring to acknowledge one another with formal bows. People in Scandinavia and northern Asia strictly limit touch to family members.

Despite these variations in customs, many cultures have produced a significant amount of artwork depicting people touching and embracing each other. This universal expression indicates that touch is an archetypal need. Children and adults alike suffer when they are not touched enough. Except for people with severe psychological problems, everybody reacts positively under the right conditions—including in public—to being touched. As long as a person does not have internal objections to being touched, due either to cultural customs or bad experiences with physical intimacy, its effects are always beneficial. Even a superficial, light touch can create a positive effect.

For those working in the fields of therapy, spa services, wellness, and healing massage, however, the therapeutic context eliminates any question of embarrassment or self-consciousness regarding touch. For these practitioners, it is a theme that has been integrated. Many others, however, remain uncomfortable with the topic. This becomes clear to me when I use the thesaurus function of my word processor to look up synonyms for the term *touch*. This function, used around the world, shows the primary associations linked to the term. The suggested synonyms cover a large spectrum that ranges from "handle" and "fondle," to "overwhelm" and "inspire." This suggests that in many people's minds, touch may be linked to acts that cause embarrassment or discomfort. However, the powerful desire of the individual to be touched is apparent in the rapidly growing interest in holistic massage methods and the return of the importance of physical connection in families and relationships.

The only synonym that to me seemed usable in the context of this book was *inspire*. The publication of this book aims to contribute to the process by which touch is recognized as something wonderful and healing, something that "inspires."

This book deals specifically with hot stone massage, which is a type of massage that is being used increasingly for relaxation, enhanced appearance, and wellness. I recommend it to you for its lively presentation, which encourages you to creatively apply the instructions and feel for yourself the power of touch and how it can be used to heal.

A healing touch, filled with love and empathy, offers access to a heightened state of consciousness and becomes a source of joy for both the one touching and the one being touched.

EVA MARIA LOHNER
Tübingen, Germany

Eva Maria Lohner, born in 1983, studied education, psychology, and sociology at Kassel and Tübingen. She works in a specialized department for the prevention of sexual violence against girls and women and is active in youth education, leading youths who want to spend a year as social volunteers. For several years she has worked as an equestrian trainer and horseback riding instructor; her work in this field has included therapeutic riding programs with disadvantaged and physically disabled youths. Eva completed her basic education in the use of healing stones with Dagmar Fleck.

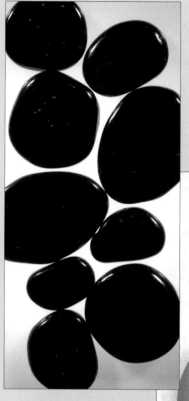

1
The Basics

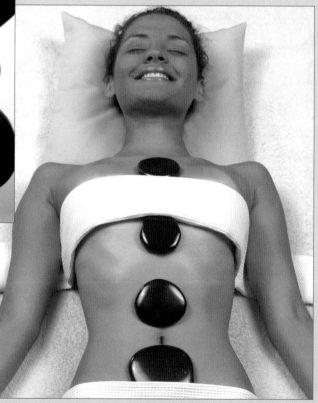

Duty makes us do things well,
But love makes us do them beautifully.

Philip Brooks

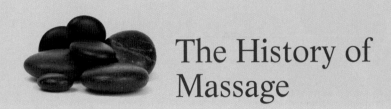

The History of Massage

THE ORIGINS OF THE WORD *massage* can be found in several different cultures. For example, the word *touch* exists in Greek as *massein,* and in Arabic as *massa.* In French we find *masser,* in Spanish *amasar* for "kneading." Hebrew uses *mashiah* to describe rubbing or anointing. At first glance, all these words describe aspects of a massage: one touches, kneads, rubs, and oils the person being massaged. However, when we look at the deeper meaning of these words, it quickly becomes clear that there are very different roots at work. Kneading is an important physiological part of massage. Kneading, however, also has a range of other associations, such as kneading dough. Likewise, touching doesn't mean simply putting one's finger on somebody. Touching is deeper, goes beyond the skin, and resurrects internal images in us. More than just lubricating the skin of the person being massaged, the act of anointing also refers to an initiation, an initiation into the feelings of both body and soul.

Over time, massage was integral to many cultures. Where it first appeared, however, remains in dispute among historians. The first detailed descriptions of massage techniques appear around 2700 BCE in China. Hippocrates (460 to about 370 BCE), the Greek doctor and

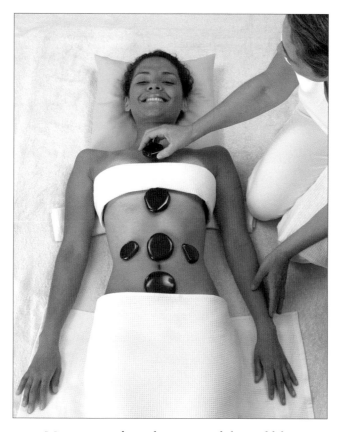

*Massage is used in cultures around the world for
both physical and spiritual healing.*

founder of scientific medicine whose oath in modified form continues
to guide doctors today, brought back knowledge of massage to Europe
from one of his journeys to Asia. The Greek philosopher and doctor
Galen (ca. 129 to 199 CE), who practiced in Rome, was one of the
most important doctors of ancient times. The teachings of Hippocrates,
which hold that illness is caused by an imbalance in bodily fluids,
experienced a renaissance in the second century CE, thanks to Galen.
Galen's in-depth studies of human anatomy led to an understanding of
the functions of body parts that influenced healing and the application
of healing massage far into the Dark Ages. Probably the best-known

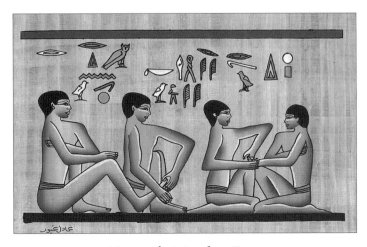

Massage depiction from Egypt

technique from that period is cupping—using hollow cups to create suction. In the ninth century Galen's writings were translated into Arabic, leading massage to a pinnacle of popularity in this culture.

Aureolus Philippus Theophrastus Bombastus von Hohenheim (1493–1541), who during his lifetime published under the pseudonym Paracelsus due to numerous disputes with other doctors, remains the namesake of many homeopathic institutions to this day. In addition to plant- and mineral-based preparations, Paracelsus successfully used gymnastic exercises and massage to heal his patients. His holis-

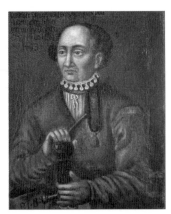

Paracelsus von Hohenheim

tic view of the human body led medicine from the Dark Ages to the Renaissance. Paracelsus wrote that a true doctor or philosopher had to be able to "turn the outside to inside" and that the "mortal shell of a person is not the actual person, only the mantle of the internal person." His thoughts had significant influence on a succession of naturopathic doctors and a decisive influence on theosophical and anthroposophical teachings.

In the seventeenth and eighteenth centuries, massage was in its heyday in France. The use of the term *massage* originated in this time period, as did many terms for classical massage techniques still in use today. *Effleurage* (stroking), *petrissage* (kneading), friction (rubbing), *tapotement* (knocking), and vibration are five techniques of classical massage that have endured from a wide range of original variations.

Aside from Asian origins, surprising levels of knowledge and skill in massage techniques existed among the native peoples of North and South America. We know that Cherokee Indians administered a type of deep tissue massage using only the index finger. By placing the index finger firmly on the spot to be treated, then vibrating it, they attained remarkable healing effects.

Whole body massages were also a part of their medical repertoire. They did not simply serve for physical relaxation but constituted holistic health maintenance. Returning conquerors brought knowledge of these practices back to Europe.

In Europe massage was practiced, but for a long time it was reduced to a purely physical type of therapy. Contemporary thought, however, is returning to a traditional holistic view. Daily bathing, body care, and hygiene, including scrubbing with warm stones, are used regularly among many native peoples to promote health. This is not just for relaxing muscles; they know that the skin is an important organ of respiration that must be kept free of sweat and dirt through regular washing, brushing, and rubbing in order to function properly.

In contrast, the physical hygiene of Europeans was dictated by moral

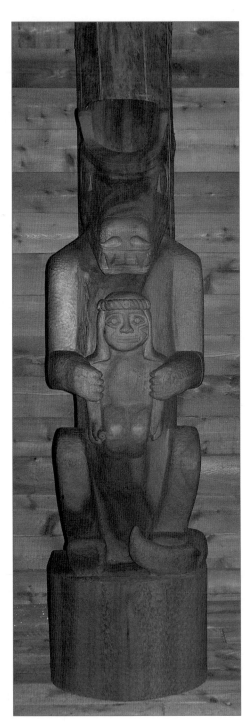

Native American medicine sculpture

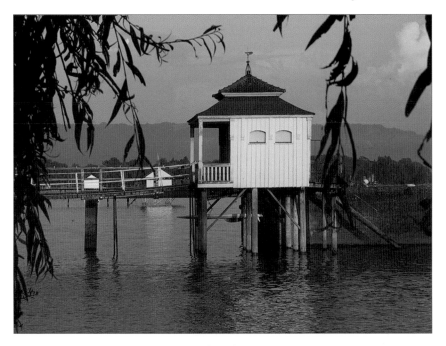

Bathing house

and social codes for centuries. While the people of the early Dark Ages still used public baths, in the seventeenth century the Catholic Church won a long-running battle against anything physically pleasurable in all classes of society. Bodily impulses were regarded as the work of the devil, and the body was the enemy of the spirit. Masseurs were careful to use strong, almost painful pressure to quash any suspicion of pleasure or violation of social mores.

He who wants to reach the source has to swim upstream.
Chinese proverb

However, during the course of the twentieth and twenty-first centuries, more specific massage techniques and variations developed in Europe that returned to treating the massage patient as a whole being.

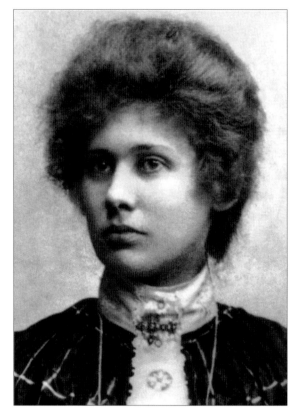

Ita Wegmann

This included the very interesting rhythmic massage developed by Dr. Ita Wegmann (1876–1943). Rhythmic massage expanded classical massage with its knowledge of anthroposophical medicine and its beliefs about innate human wisdom.

Anthroposophical medicine treats the individual as a whole being. The word's roots come from the Greek *anthropos,* meaning "human," and *sophia,* meaning "wisdom." The goal of anthroposophical medicine is not to remove symptoms but to explore what might be causing the illness, whether it is emanating from social surroundings or the spiritual and mental needs of the patient. To this end, a number of elements were added to the massage technique: for example, deep tissue massage,

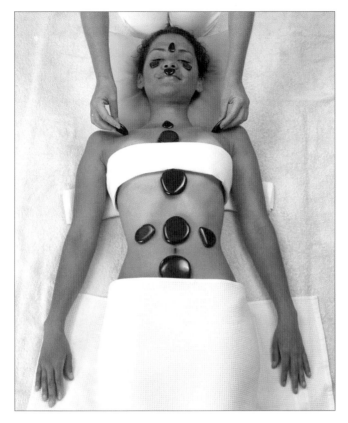

Hot stone massage

rhythmic sequences, and various forms of the *lemniscate,* or infinity symbol. The goal of the massage is to create connections and to reach the soul of a person via physical work on the body.

Today there is a broad spectrum of massage available, especially in the area of holistic massage, where there are many important variations. To focus not only on physical conditions, but to view the person as a whole—a unit of body, soul, understanding, and spirit—is the aim of our work. For us, massage, aside from its beneficial physical relaxation, also stimulates the life force energy. In this book, we want to introduce you to a holistic modality that is spreading across the globe due to its beneficial effects: massage using hot stones.

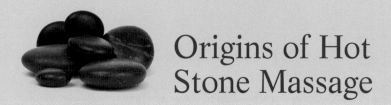

Origins of Hot Stone Massage

TWO TYPES OF MASSAGE USING HOT STONES are currently practiced widely: LaStone and hot stone. The roots of both these types of massage reach back over two millennia. They were known in Chinese medicine, as well as among Hawaiian and Native American shamans. In Asia, records show that a type of therapy using hot stones was used even before the birth of Christ. The origin of massage with hot stones is most likely rooted in ancient Nepal, Tibet, or western China, where people ascribed a secret, special, and invisible healing power to stones. Aside from invisible healing powers, stones have useful physical characteristics. For example, their ability to store warmth or cold makes them helpful in alleviating a wide range of ailments.

The LaStone massage combines classic massage techniques with the healing knowledge of North American Hopi Indians. This type of massage was revived and refined in the 1990s through the work of masseuse Mary Nelson, the founder of LaStone therapy.

LaStone therapy utilizes fifty-four black basalt (lava) stones and eighteen white marble stones; the basalt stones are heated in water to a temperature of 122°F (50°C) or higher, while the marble rocks are cooled on ice. The focus of the work is the heated stones, with the cold

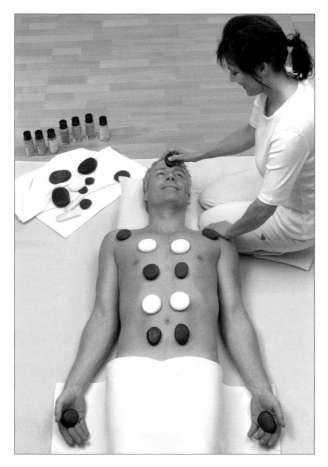

LaStone therapy

marble stones applied as a counterbalance. Warm-cold stimulation creates tension in the body, which causes the body to attempt to rebalance itself. Much as in the application of Sebastian Kneipp's hydrotherapy (the Kneipp Cure), this stimulates the metabolism and strengthens blood vessels. LaStone is a trademark and may be used only by authorized providers.

In contrast, the application of hot stone massage, which has its origins in Hawaii, is not trademarked. It is open to everyone and allows the therapist a less restrictive way of working with heated

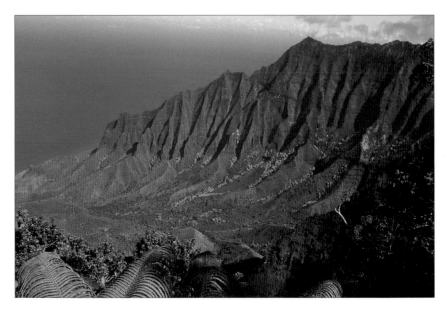

Hawaii

stones. In Hawaiian, hot stone massage is called *pohaku* (rock/stone) *wai* (water) *ola* (life, health, being healthy).

Since ancient times, the people of Hawaii have used heated stones for physical and spiritual healing. The island inhabitants developed a very effective massage using smooth volcanic rocks as tools. Massage with heated stones loosens muscles and relieves tension, pleasantly stimulating circulation and warmth throughout the body, and calming the soul. The wellness massage with hot stones is appreciated by both therapists—for whom it makes the work easier—and clients, who are able to enjoy the relaxing and revitalizing effect of the stones from the very first moment of the treatment.

Hot stone massage deliberately uses primarily gentle, noninvasive stimulation. Cold stones are usually not used, since the massage avoids very strong contrast. In his book *Aurum Manus* the well-known masseur Ricky Welch nicely formulates the stimulation law of massage:

The Stimulation Law of Massage

Gentle stimulation stimulates.
Stronger stimulation increases vitality.
Strong stimulation blocks.
Strongest stimulation harms.
Remember: be stingy with stimulation!

This stimulation law also applies to massage with hot stones. A key element of this massage is to proceed carefully and with empathy. Sometimes less is more!

Today, hot stone massage has become a trend in beauty treatments, wellness, and massage. This is because of its various uses, the most prominent of which is its high value in relaxation and increased overall well-being.

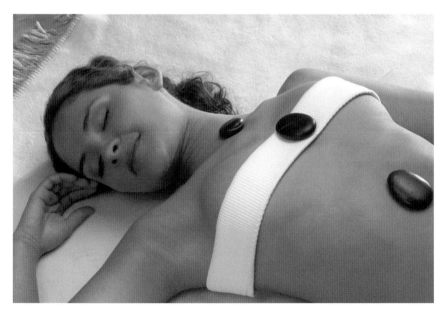

Hot stone massage is valued in large part for its relaxing effects.

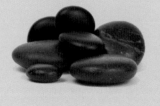

Application Areas and Effects of Hot Stone Massage

HOT STONE MASSAGE HAS BROAD APPLICATION, with a wide range of effects. It is based on a comprehensive activation of body processes, and there is almost no aspect of the organism that is not affected by this type of massage. Its most important application areas are as follows:

- Improves circulation
- Strengthens lymph flow
- Improves soft tissue metabolism
- Removes toxins
- Alleviates muscle tension
- Can be used for joint problems, back pain, and sore muscles
- Has a calming effect
- Alleviates tension caused by stress and its effects (for example, headaches, insomnia, digestive problems)
- Strengthens the immune system

This short list includes the main benefits of hot stone massage, but

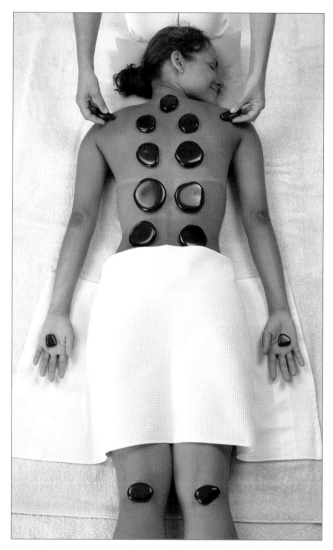

Hot stone massage has a wide range of beneficial effects.

not all of its possibilities. The combination of the deep power of the stones, the warmth of the treatment, and the massage calms, relaxes, and increases the metabolism of the body tissue. This particularly benefits types of tissue that usually have slow metabolism, for example, tendons, ligaments, and connective tissue. At the same time, the treatment increases the flexibility of these tissues and the mobility of the joints. It also causes the blood vessels to dilate, which leads to improved circulation. This in turn leads to increased oxygen, nutrients, and antibodies, and a surge in cell production. The lymph flow and immune system are stimulated, increasing the removal of toxins. Muscle tension is released and pain alleviated. Moreover, remarkable effects have been observed among people who suffer from chronically cold hands and feet. This is due to the positive influence of this application on our energy distribution system, which we know as the Triple Warmer meridian in Chinese medicine. On the spiritual, mental, and soul level, hot stone massage encourages the resolution of energetic blockages, and causes a deep releasing and relaxing. Nerves that are sensitive to the touch are stimulated over a broad area, the autonomic nervous system is soothed, and traces of stress are washed from the body.

Caution! In the presence of acute illness, massage should be administered only by experienced therapists, since it is possible to unknowingly do more harm than good. Moreover, hot stone massage should not replace treatment by a doctor or healing practitioner, although it can support such treatment. If in doubt, discuss the use of this massage with your doctor or therapist.

When Should You Not Use Hot Stone Massage?

Since massage exerts such a strong influence on the energy body, under certain circumstances it is not advised. Conditions precluding massage include infections accompanied by fever, contagious diseases, infectious skin diseases, skin rashes, burns, and wounds that have not yet healed. Moreover, caution is needed immediately after surgery, in the case of thrombosis, vein infections, and large varicose veins. Areas above bruises, infected injuries, or freshly healed bone fractures should not be massaged directly.

In the case of pregnancy, severe heart problems, tumors, or during chemotherapy, massage should be carried out only after consulting with your doctor.

Other than that, the regular application of hot stone massage has a very positive effect on overall well-being. The beneficial effects of the therapy, however, are not limited to physical conditions; they also help us to regain or maintain mental balance. This is accomplished by including the body's meridians and chakras in the treatment.

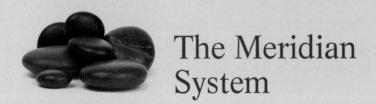

The Meridian System

MORE THAN 2,000 YEARS AGO Chinese medicine first described the system of the meridians. The meridian system consists of twelve main meridians, which comprise six meridian pairs, which in turn are assigned to the five transformation phases of Chinese medicine—our energetic connection to fire, earth, metal, water, and wood—not to be confused with the four natural elements of Western culture (fire, earth, air, and water). Whereas the Western elements are static components that describe the composition of the world, the transformation phases describe a dynamic, transforming, and developing world. In relation to our health, this means that we can remain healthy, or improve our health, when we adjust to external conditions and are able to change in harmony with natural cycles. The view that health is a static condition, occasionally interrupted by illness, is alien to traditional Chinese doctors.

Each of the main meridians—mirror images that run along both sides of the body—is linked to an internal organ, with one of each meridian pair linked to a hollow organ (yang meridian) and the other linked to a storage organ (yin meridian).

Overview of the Transformation Phases and Meridian Pairs		
TRANSFORMATION PHASE	**MERIDIAN PAIR**	
	Yin meridian	**Yang meridian**
Wood	Liver	Gall Bladder
Fire I	Heart	Small Intestine
Fire II	Pericardium	Triple Warmer
Earth	Spleen, pancreas	Stomach
Metal	Lung	Large Intestine
Water	Kidney	Bladder

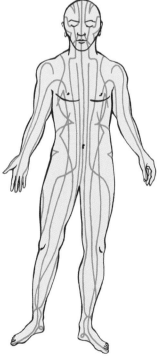

The meridian system

In addition to connections between the meridians and internal organs, there are connections to other body parts, as well as to sensory perceptions and spiritual experiences. For example, the Lung meridian corresponds not only to the storage organ of the lungs but also to all body parts related to breathing, such as nose, throat, larynx, bronchia, and, of course, skin. The related sensory perception is the sense of smell. Exchange and communication are the spiritual experiences linked to the Lung meridian, which is easy to understand since the air we all breathe links us to our fellow human beings.

The partner of the Lung meridian is the Large Intestine meridian. Partner meridians support each other in the case of disturbances but can also negatively affect each other if long-term blockages exist. It is well known that the lungs have a close relationship to the large intestine. If a body is overburdened, the lungs attempt, via the mucous membranes, to remove more toxins. This is why intestinal problems are often accompanied by breathing problems.

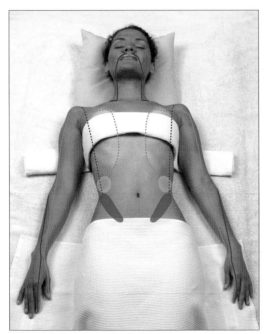

The Lung and Large Intestine partner meridians with their internal branches.

The function of the meridians is to create a whole network among the organs, joints, and other parts of the body, such as the skin, bones, muscles, and tendons. In addition, the meridians ensure a balance between the yin and yang aspects of the organs. In Chinese medicine, yin and yang refer to any type of contrast. All of life, including our bodies and emotions, is understood as a rhythm of sound and silence, day and night, warm and cold, activity and rest. Yang character is everything that is light, outwardly focused, active, masculine. Yin character is dark, internally focused, steady, feminine. Yin and yang are like fire and water, controlling each other. Fire can evaporate water; water can douse fire. A harmonious interplay between these two components maintains or engenders a healthy organism.

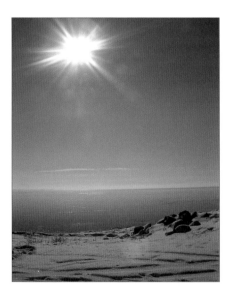

Fire and water, the balance of life

The terms *yin* and *yang* do not indicate anything about the energetic condition of a meridian. Every meridian can have a lack or excess of either yin or yang. A lack of yang is expressed by fatigue and cold; an excess of yang manifests as heat and redness. Insufficient yin is indicated by dryness and heat; too much yin manifests as excessive interior dampness.

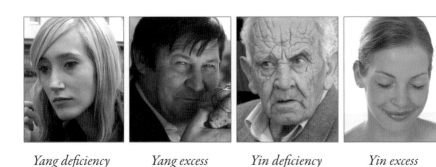

| *Yang deficiency* | *Yang excess* | *Yin deficiency* | *Yin excess* |

Every metabolic process, every thought, and every emotion leads to the consumption or production of certain energies. Thus, rhythmic activity in different areas of bodily function leads to either energy consumption or energy release. Meridians can be seen as the energy pathways of the body, through which released energy is distributed via fine ion streams. In this way, excess and scarcity are balanced to maintain equilibrium in the energetic whole. These ion streams always take the path of least resistance, usually traveling along muscles, tendons, bones, or blood vessels, and only occasionally passing through them. The transition from one meridian to the next occurs in a regular exchange on the chest, hand, head, or foot. Through fingers and toes we exchange energy with our surroundings.

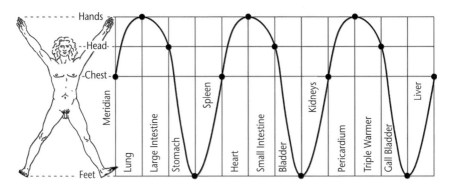

Energy flow of the meridians in the body

The meridian system is highly sensitized. This explains why smog, electromagnetic frequencies, and other disturbances have a negative influence on our biological and energetic whole.

During massage with hot stones the meridian pathways are gently activated or balanced. Imagine your body as a land crossed by rivers (meridians), rivers that have no dams, marshes, or dry zones. If your holistic system is "flowing well" and all your regions are sufficiently "watered," your life energy (Chinese *chi*) is increased and your quality of life enhanced.

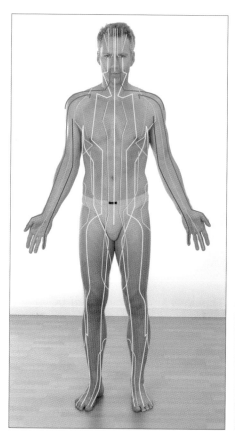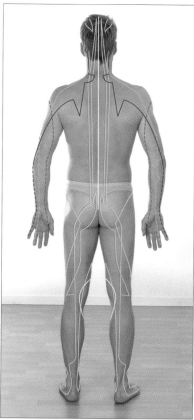

The body's meridians

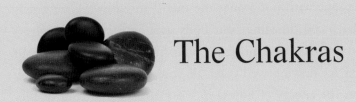

The Chakras

"I have been in outer space many times," bragged the astronaut, "but I have seen neither God nor angels."

"And I have operated on many smart brains," answered the brain researcher, "but nowhere have I found even a single thought."

Sophie's World

JUST AS THOUGHTS ARE INVISIBLE, chakras and the aura can be equally elusive. Even though we usually cannot see thoughts, everyone will confirm that they exist. Some may even suggest being able to read the thoughts of others. Expressions such as, "I just thought the same thing," or, "I know exactly what you mean" are known to each of us. It is similar with the chakras. Being able to visually perceive chakras and auras is not, as is often claimed, a special skill of particularly perceptive people. We all have the ability to perceive fine energies, although for the most part we are not aware of this ability. If we want to integrate this ability

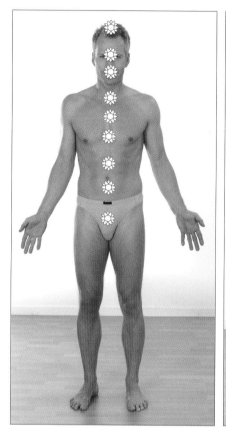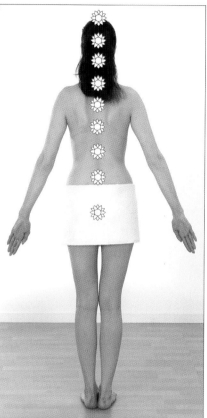

Locations of the nine chakras used in hot stone massage

back into our lives, we simply need to learn a few simple techniques to sensitize our perception. As with many things in life, all it takes is practice.

Origin of Chakra Teachings

The description of the chakras as we know them today originates in India. From the old Indian cultural language Sanskrit, which has been spoken since about 1500 BCE, comes the name *chakra,* which roughly translates into "wheel" or "circle." Similar observations and descriptions of fine-substance energies that surround the human body are also found in Native American and European traditions. While the thoughts at first seem very different, when examined more closely they complement each other and form a unified picture.

In recent European history, the chakras were first described in theosophy. The landmark work *The Chakra,* by Charles W. Leadbeater, was written in 1899 but wasn't published until 1927, in London and Adyar (India). Theosophy has existed since ancient times, and the theosophic worldview of pantheism—that God is everything and everywhere—has reappeared in different eras. Today's theosophy is based primarily on the work of Madame Blavatsky (1831–1891), who was in contact with Tibetan masters and founded the Theosophical Society, which has been meeting in India since 1882. Rudolf Steiner belonged to this society for some time before he founded his own school of thought, which he called anthroposophism.

Madame Blavatsky's goal was to create the preconditions for a world religion in which all faiths have justification for existence, and each individual is able to study the different teachings and allow them to coexist. From our point of view, this is a very wise approach and one

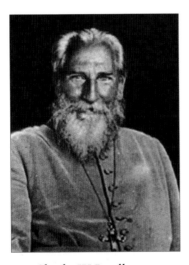

Charles W. Leadbeater

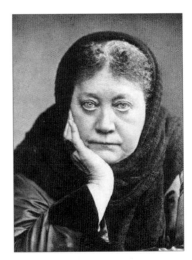

Madame Blavatsky

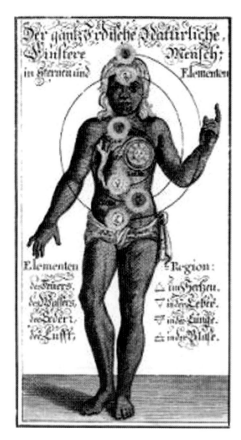

Theosophic chakra depiction

that in earlier times, during the Renaissance, was promoted by philosophers, theosophists, natural scientists, mystics, doctors, and astrologers alike.

Nonetheless, theosophical teaching is not the only truth, as Madame Blavatsky acknowledged during her lifetime: "It requires the proper perception of objective facts to finally discover that the only true world is a subjective one."

This subjective viewpoint is also reflected in the theosophic representation of the chakras, in which the original nine body-specific chakras were reduced to seven. The number of chakras differs in various other records, as well. Tibetan systems, for example, describe three, five, or six chakras; Indian systems, six, seven, or nine; and

European and Native American systems, nine or ten. At first glance, this may seem contradictory, but upon careful examination it becomes clear that although each system describes all fundamental characteristics and qualities of the chakras, some philosophies group together several chakras as *units*. This is often the case with the root and sacral chakras, sacral and solar plexus chakras, heart and thymus chakras, nose and brow chakras, and brow and crown chakras. This is most apparent in Tibetan teachings, where the system of three chakras is used in the context of the trinity of the Buddha body (brow), speech (throat), and spirit (heart). Yet five chakras are used when they are differentiated by activity (root chakra), characteristics (sacral chakra), spirit (heart chakra), speech (throat chakra), and body function (brow chakra). Oftentimes, mention is also made of a sixth chakra, the crown chakra, which in Tibetan teaching is important when leaving the body during the dying process.

The number of chakras in the different systems does not refer to how many chakras actually exist, but rather which (and thus how many) chakras play a role in reference to a specific system or context. This

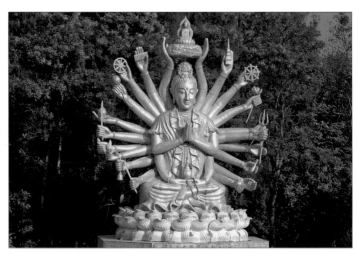

Buddha statue with ten pairs of raised arms, corresponding to the symbolic significance of the ten chakras in the Indian system

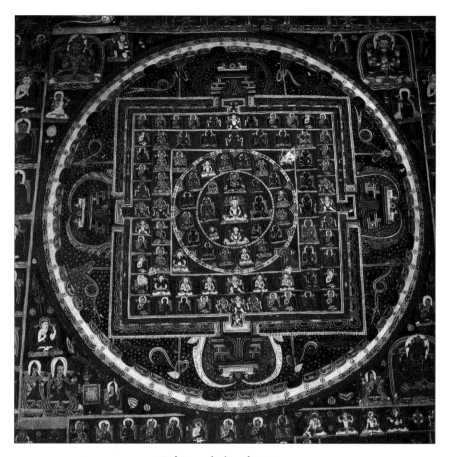

Tibetan chakra depiction

explains the variation in number of chakras, ranging from three to ten.

In theosophy, seven planets—Sun, Moon, Mercury, Venus, Mars, Jupiter, and Saturn—are the central system of reference. Astrology and many other scientific areas reference this group of seven. For this reason, only seven chakras are mentioned in the context of this teaching. The Indian chakra system commonly uses nine chakras, which in addition to the seven planets listed above also references the rising (Rahu) and waning (Ketu) moon nodes. Moon nodes are those points in the sky where the paths of the sun and moon intersect. They are referenced in astrology in the same way planets are used for horoscopes and other

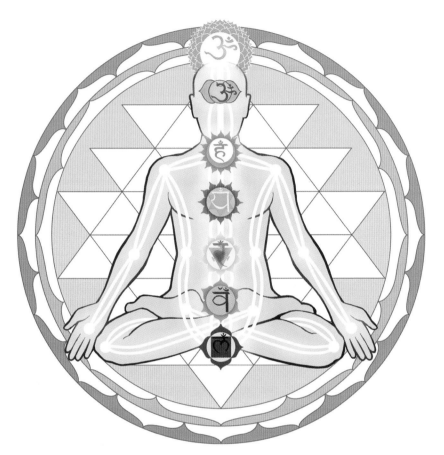

Chakra depiction in the Vedic system

purposes. Since Rahu and Ketu are considered "difficult" points, they are often ignored, and with them their corresponding chakras, thymus (Rahu) and nose (Ketu).

North Indian chakra systems do not value individual chakras differently; none is better or worse, or more or less spiritual than another. For this reason, in many transmissions of Indian chakra teachings we find references to all nine body-specific chakras, as well as a tenth chakra outside the physical body (one hand width above the head). This is similar to non-Christian European teachings. While these teachings assign the nine chakras to the three worlds—Asgard (upper

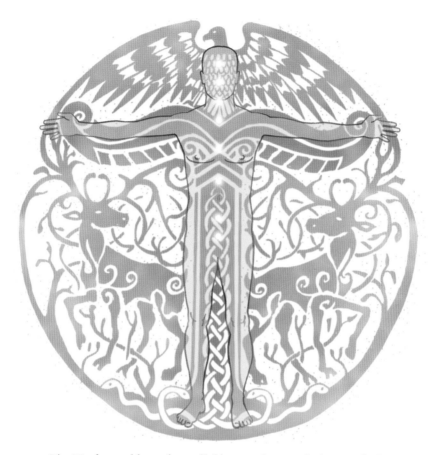

The Nordic world tree (tree of life) as it relates to the human body

world/head), Midgard (middle world/chest), and Utgard (lower world/ stomach)—the value assignment of good or bad (heaven, earth, and hell) to these three worlds only occurred in Christianity. Until then they had been considered to be of equal value, as reflected in the oldest Edda (Nordic) poems in the second stanza of the first song (the *Völuspá*): "Nine worlds I knew, the nine in the tree, / With mighty roots, beneath the mold." This description of the "world tree" mirrored both the universe and human nature.

In hot stone massage, we include all nine body-specific chakras into our treatment, simply because they exist and because in more than twenty years of research and healing, we have had very good experiences using them. Treatment of the neglected thymus and nose chakras has particularly effective consequences for physical health, spiritual and mental orientation, and freedom of mind.

The fact that even people who see auras often don't recognize these two chakras may have cultural origins. After puberty the thymus gland usually recedes and turns into fatty tissue. However, it remains an important organ of our immune system. A light tapping on the thymus region causes us to feel strong and brave—we know this from the example of the great apes. However, strength, courage, and conviction are not qualities that are in demand in today's world. After all, much is done to foster a population that cowers, functions, works hard, and is easily manipulated. Interestingly, Indian yogis and sadhus, who have the ability to control their own bodies and direct healing processes, have fully intact thymus glands.

The reason the nose chakra is often not recognized is linked on the one hand to its clear, ethereal light (like the shimmer of air above hot earth) and on the other to our hardly being able to "have a nose for" something in today's world. Too many impressions confuse our sense of smell, often paralyzing this instinct altogether. In light of this background, we find it all the more important to include these two chakras in our work.

What Are Chakras?

In different cultures and holistic healing methods, the human body is seen as a cycle of flowing energies. Chakras, however, are not only intersection points along the center of the body where the different energy cycles meet but also can be viewed as surrounding fields with bodylike contours, in which the first chakra, the root chakra, is at the same time the smallest and innermost body, similar to the Russian matryoshka dolls pictured on page 33.

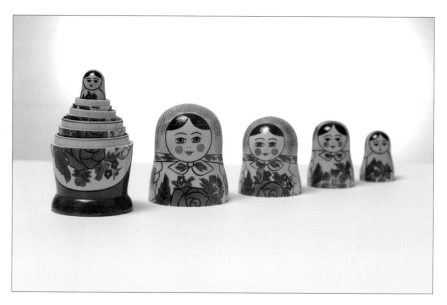

Russian nesting dolls as an analogy for the chakras

The first and smallest body is about the size of a hand, the second surrounds the first and is a few inches larger, the third surrounds the second, and so on until we reach the ninth chakra, or body, which roughly corresponds to the size of the physical body. Each of these bodies can be viewed as an individual person, with its own way of thinking, feeling, and acting. If we move our consciousness into one of these bodies, we suddenly see the world in a very specific way. For example, in the sacral chakra we are especially interested in our relationship to the world; in the heart chakra, fulfillment through the world; and in the throat chakra, communication with the world. We then act accordingly. The "focal point" of our consciousness is always located in the head of the respective body, which is where descriptions localize the position of the chakra. It is at this point that the respective body is easiest to influence. In its fullness, however, it is not confined to this particular spot, which we often feel very clearly in chakra treatments.

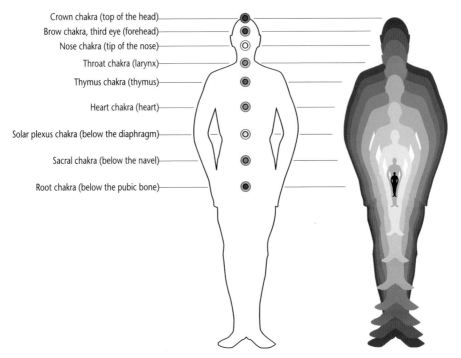

Crown chakra (top of the head)
Brow chakra, third eye (forehead)
Nose chakra (tip of the nose)
Throat chakra (larynx)
Thymus chakra (thymus)
Heart chakra (heart)
Solar plexus chakra (below the diaphragm)
Sacral chakra (below the navel)
Root chakra (below the pubic bone)

The chakras as energetic bodies

The Significance of the Chakras

Surprisingly, the characteristics and significance of the chakras are largely the same in different cultural teachings.

- The root chakra ensures our survival. It is the driving force in our lives. It is here that the sexual drive in a reproductive context is located.
- In the sacral chakra, too, we find the theme of sexuality, albeit on a different plane. This relates more to relationship and partnership, contact and affection for the other.
- The solar plexus chakra affects our expression in acts and deeds and our feeling of self-worth as a mirror of our position in the world.

• The heart chakra is the center of our feelings and steers our desire for fulfillment. Themes such as empathy and understanding are localized here.

• The thymus chakra has qualities that affect our ability to accept responsibility and live according to personal convictions.

• The throat chakra is the seat of our ability to communicate, to engage in verbal exchange and make connections.

• The nose chakra is the seat of our instincts and intuition. This affects our ability to judge situations clearly.

• The brow chakra contains our intuition and powers of imagination. It is here that one realizes whether she is staying true to her life's course.

• The crown chakra expresses our life areas as inspiration or as nightly dreams. It is linked to the original intent of our being. Native American teachings refer to the dream body, and contend that we are on the earth to dance our dreams into being.

Thus each chakra has a creative center in which we create and maintain certain aspects of our lives, as well as recognize and dissolve them. It is possible to build something new in one part of our lives, while we dissolve or complete something in another part of our lives. "Building" and "dissolving" cause different energy movement in the corresponding chakras. In the case of creative, building processes, we note a turn to the right (clockwise, observed from the outside), while dissolving processes cause a turn to the left (counterclockwise, observed from the outside). These turning movements give the chakras their names, from the Sanskrit, where chakra means "wheel." Both movements are necessary for our being, and one is neither better nor worse than the other (see image on page 36). Only the balance of construction and dissolution enable a stable existence (think of digestion = construction, and

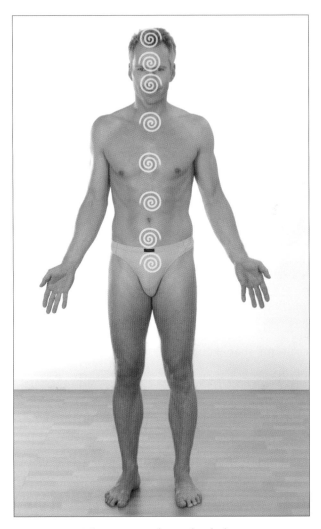

The energy cycles in the chakras

excretion = dissolution). For this reason, traditional Chinese doctors often say, "Life is change—stagnation is death."

Treating the Chakras

Blockages in the chakras cannot be diagnosed by the direction of the chakra movement, whether it is turning left or right, since this only indicates that something is forming and dissolving in each area of life. Rather, blockages indicate that the process has slowed down or even stopped altogether and that the chakra is turning very slowly, or hardly at all. The warming stones of hot stone massage stimulate the chakras in their movement without manipulating the direction of the movement in any way. This improves the flow of energy, which activates and eases the respective process in life. The placing of warm stones automatically has the greatest effect where it is most needed, where the movement of energy is experiencing the most difficulty. Hot stones have the least influence on chakras with free-flowing energy. In this way, the placing of warm stones is diagnosis and treatment in one. As long as we don't overdo the treatment by placing

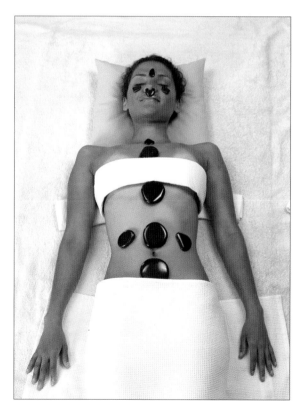

Chakra treatment using hot stones

stones that are too hot or keeping them in place for too long, usually a hot stone massage will gently stimulate and balance the chakras.

Since each chakra contains spiritual aspects (goals and aims), mental aspects (views and ideas), aspects of the soul (feelings and experiences), and aspects of the body (control and regulation impulses), a chakra balancing treatment has a holistic effect on spirit, mind, understanding, and body, resulting in their being in harmony with one another. From an energy perspective, hot stone massage leads not only to harmony of energy within a chakra but also to harmony in the energy exchange among different chakras. We experience this as an increase in strength and ability, as well as an increase in confidence and freedom. And we experience the reflection of those changes in our lives, since each change in one chakra necessarily leads to changes in life and experiences.

Choosing the Chakra Gems

As a conclusion to many hot stone massages, we place room-temperature chakra gems on the body. In all our courses, trainings, and practice, we have had our best experiences using an intuitive choice of these stones along with the traditional Indian order. Choosing the chakra gems in an analytical way is much more complex than simply assigning the color of a stone to the respective color of a chakra. For example, different stones of the same family can have effects on different chakras. This is because stones have a type of aura color that corresponds better with the fine-substance energy of the chakras than with the visible color of the stone. For example, if you have ten rock crystals in front of you, each may have a different aura color. Analytically, this would demand that we compare the specific effects of each individual stone with the themes of the different chakras; only then could we begin to approach the best correspondence. While this is an interesting process, it is also a long and complicated one. Therefore we find it more practical to proceed by intuition,

Chakra	Stone		Description
Crown	Amethyst		Spirituality, meditation, intuition, stimulates conscious perception and is good for headaches
Brow	Lapis lazuli		Knowledge, power, helps one to be master of his own domain and to find the right path
Nose	Rock crystal		Clarity, neutrality, stimulates the flow of energy, improves perception
Throat	Blue chalcedony		Good for lymph flow, communication, self-expression
Thymus	Jasper		Increases courage, makes one more dynamic, brings energy and increases resistance
Heart	Rose quartz		Strengthens the heart, increases the ability to recognize deep emotions, increases empathy
Solar plexus	Amber		Good for stomach, spleen and liver, strengthens belief in oneself, sunny disposition
Sacral	Jade/Nephrite		Increases ability to be in relationships, enhances power of understanding and decision making
Root	Ruby/Garnet		Stimulates circulation, adrenal glands, and sexual organs; represents passion and joy of life

a resonance method (for example, a dowsing rod), or kinesiology tests.

If you have difficulty with intuitive correspondence, the table above suggests stones that may be effective in addressing the themes of the

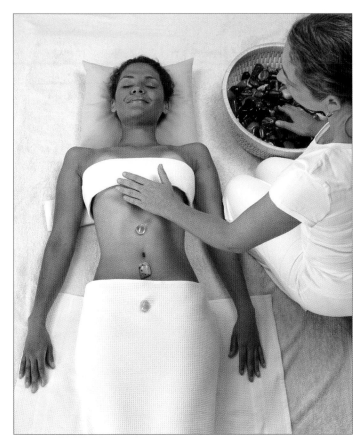

Intuitive choice of chakra gems and crystals

different chakras. Again, this is merely an approximation that may not apply in all cases. The chapter titled Gemstone Chakra Treatment in part 4 mentions additional stones that are well suited for this purpose and that have proved to be effective via the intuitive selection process.

These stones are primarily balancing, harmonizing stones. But be careful in your work and be guided by your own feelings and intuition. If you think a particular stone is not suitable, choose one that feels better to you. As with the meridians, you are working with a highly sensitive system, and this demands sensitivity in your work.

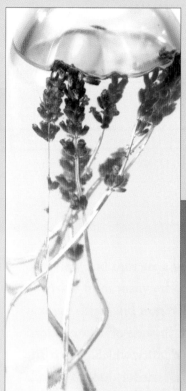

2
Materials

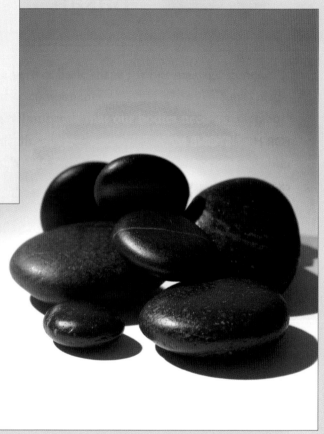

Things only have the value we give them.

Molière

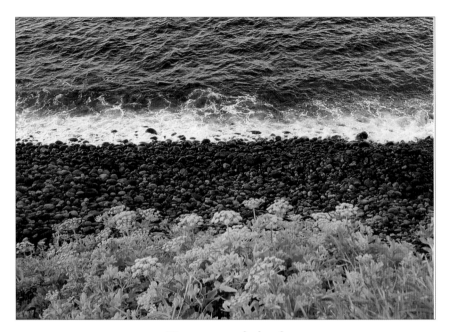

Hot stones on the beach

frequencies resonate in the human body. Visualize the effects of the stones as music that is good for us, and to which we enjoy listening. Our bodies vibrate to this rhythm. On another fine-substance level, the body (or bodies—see the chapter on chakras) vibrates to the "music" of the stones.

The following healing effects result from the composition of basalt.

Color

Just as black absorbs all light, black stones have a receptive quality. They help to absorb excess energy and can be used effectively in the treatment of pain. Black is relaxing on all levels and

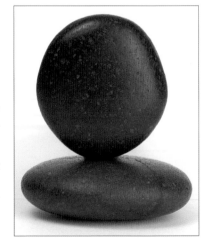

Black basalt stones

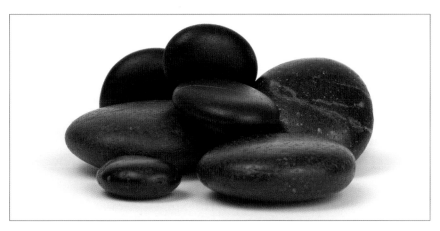

*Selection of basalt stones showing subtle variations in color
due to the different concentrations of minerals*

helps us to remain centered and able to concentrate on our own internal light of being.

Minerals

Silica strengthens body tissue and hair, skin, and nails. It supports various immune reactions in bodily fluids and is important in guarding against frequent illness. Silica reduces infection, supports the healing of wounds, prevents the formation of scars, and slows the aging process. It helps repair feelings of exhaustion and excess sensitivity and creates an internal feeling of well-being. Silica transmits stability and security.

Calcium stimulates the production and constitution of tissue, bones, and teeth. Calcium plays an important role in the transmission of impulses from nerves to organs and muscles and has a positive effect on the activity of the heart. It supports and balances physical, spiritual, and mental development processes, stabilizing and providing internal energy.

Magnesium resolves cramps, relaxes muscles, and helps resolve migraines and tension-induced headaches. It increases blood circulation, improves the performance of the heart, and prevents tissue and arteries from becoming clogged. Magnesium has a calming effect and increases resistance to stress. It transmits a happy, optimistic approach to life.

Iron is necessary for the creation of hemoglobin and red blood cells. Iron increases the oxygen content in muscles and organs, which supports their vitality. Iron strengthens the immune system and our willpower and ability to get our way.

Creation

Basalt is one of the so-called primary stones, because it is created directly from liquid lava. Primary stones increase our ability to discover our own internal potential. They bring recognition of our undiscovered capacities.

Much as the mineral ingredients in liquid lava determine which mineral is formed as a result, primary stones help to determine our predispositions—what is contained within ourselves that should be developed or lived more amply. Since volcanic stones are created comparatively quickly, basalt supports us in quickly actualizing the potential it helps us to discover.

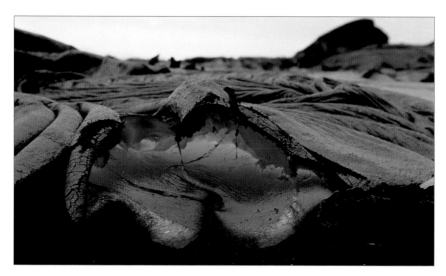

Lava flow in Hawaii

Crystal Structures

Mineralogy differentiates among eight different crystal structures that result from the internal atomic makeup of minerals, which become apparent in the external appearance of crystals. These crystal structures are based on the seven geometric forms: square (cubic), hexagonal, rectangular (tetragonal), triangle (trigonal), rhombus, parallelogram (monoklin), and trapezoid (triklin). Rare exceptions are several minerals without a regular internal structure, referred to as *amorphous*. In stone-healing lore, crystal structures reflect what we perceive and create in our lives—how we live, through what lens we see the world. A lifestyle could be characterized by emotions, perceptions, moods, and emotional actions; or by reason, knowledge, mental strength, analytical thinking, and rationality. For example, if one person lives a life characterized by a high degree of order, we call this a cubic, or square, lifestyle. The amorphous lifestyle describes the exact opposite, a life in which personal freedom and impulsiveness play a big role. In this way, each crystal structure characterizes specific character traits and habits.

Basalt cannot be assigned to a clear crystal structure, because it is a stone comprised of different minerals. Interestingly, however, we most frequently find three structures—rhombus, monoklin, and triklin—that affect themes of the emotional area, as opposed to the more rational cubic, hexagonal, and tetragonal structures. The structures that exist in basalt, therefore, not only help us to relax deeply and release but also support the ability to experience a deep internal connection with both self and others. Basalt helps us to recognize our own interests and desires and strengthens our ability to pursue them. It helps to develop our lighter senses and gives us the strength to rely on our intuition.

Thus, we once again complete a circle. A circle of the massage application with warm stones is beneficial in and of itself, and the energetic effects of basalt are beneficial from a stone-healing perspective.

Locations

The islands of Hawaii were created by volcanic activity in the Pacific Ocean. Hawaii is far removed from any continental landmass, meaning that the islands have to weather the strong Pacific winds without any protection. Over the course of thousands of years, the winds and rain have smoothed and polished the basalt stones found here. For this reason, stones originating here are almost completely smooth and well-suited for massage purposes.

Original Hawaiian hot stones are completely natural, collected by hand, and come from one of the most beautiful and spiritual places in the world. Anyone who has ever been to Hawaii knows the beautiful beaches, majestic mountains, clear blue water, and the great *aloha* spirit of these islands.

There are many massage techniques and a wide variety of stones that can be used in hot stone massage. Although some stones are offered as Hawaiian basalt, they may have other origins. A large proportion of available stones are manufactured in Chinese factories. As long as it is indeed

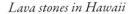

Lava stones in Hawaii

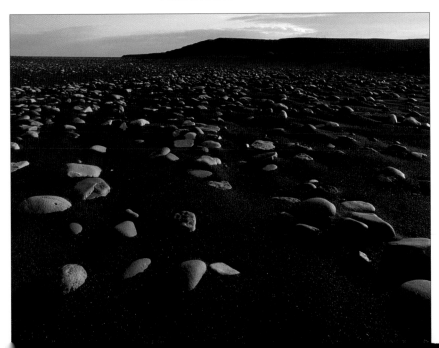

basalt, these stones will work in the same way. However, because many hot stones are used outside the natural stone or mineral trade sectors, there are a number of other types of stones in circulation. Dark volcanic stones of similar density are acceptable for the purpose of massage, as well as the deep stone *gabbroid* that comes from the same magma that forms basalt lava when it reaches Earth's surface. Unfortunately, however, production is also often "supplemented" in dishonest ways. If, for example, the water in your warming apparatus takes on a black color after the initial application, you can be sure that you do not have original Hawaiian hot stones or similar stones made from real basalt. It is always a good idea to buy hot stones from a vendor you trust.

Moreover, basalt occurs around the world, making imitations completely unnecessary. Natural basalt stones similar to those from Hawaii can be found, for example, in the Canary Islands, Iceland, and southern Italy; on the east coast of Australia; and in many other volcanic regions around the world. Beautiful, naturally smooth basalt can also be found

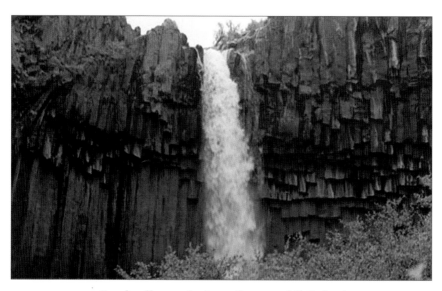

Basalt pillars at the Svartifoss waterfall, Iceland
(Photo by A. Partz)

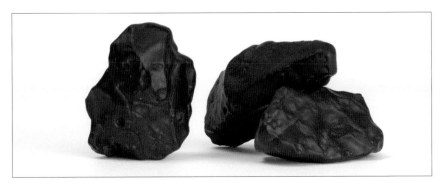

Argentine basalt (ventifaz)

on the southernmost tip of Argentina in Patagonia. The native population here calls the stones *ventifaz,* which roughly translates into "wind faces." These stones, however, have a somewhat irregular surface and are thus better suited for being placed on the body rather than for actual massage.

A safe alternative to naturally shaped stones can be domestic basalt that is smoothed and polished.

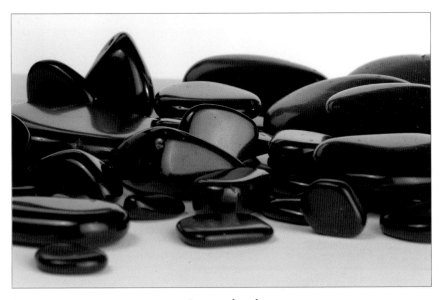

German basalt

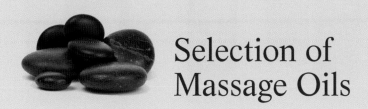

Selection of Massage Oils

THE EFFECTIVENESS OF HOT STONE MASSAGE depends on the skill and internal disposition of the person carrying out the massage, the quality of the stones, and the selection and quality of the massage oil.

Oil is nourishing and detoxifying for the body. It affects the internal organs by being absorbed through the skin. For massage, choose an oil that corresponds to the senses of the person being massaged; it should feel good on the skin, and the client should be able to smell it clearly. For hot stone massage we suggest a generally well-received, gentle oil such as sweet almond, jojoba, macadamia nut, or olive oil. A relaxing, calming, balancing, and lightening effect can be attained by adding St. John's wort oil or evening primrose oil (about one-third of the total) to the oils named above.

It is important to use high-quality oil from specialty stores that carry organic wellness products (see page 64 for specific recommendations and massage oil recipes). Oil should be cold-pressed—ideally from the first pressing, and, as far as possible, pure (without the addition of other ingredients). Only in this way can you be sure that the oil contains all its vitamins and minerals.

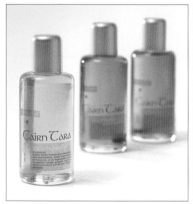
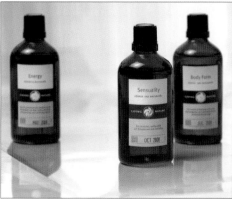

High-quality massage oil

Almond Oil

The seeds for the production of oil come from the stone fruits of sweet almond trees. Almond oil is one of the classic oils of antiquity and was a veritable treasure in those times. It is characterized by being particularly mild, easily absorbed, rich in vitamin E, and extremely well suited to clarifying skin tone and alleviating dry skin. Sweet almond oil nourishes and protects the skin, leaving it smooth and soft, and reduces irritation in sensitive areas. Since it is absorbed slowly, it allows for gliding strokes, making it an excellent massage oil. However, as a precaution, almond oil should not be used on people who are allergic to nuts.

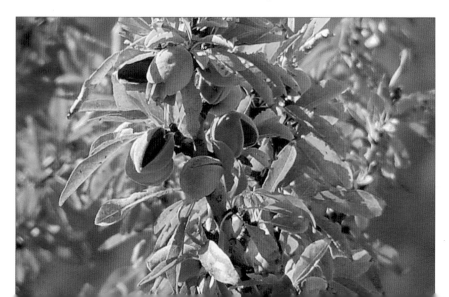

Jojoba Oil

The difference between jojoba and other oils lies in jojoba being more of a liquid wax than an oil. Jojoba oil is pressed from the nut of a bush that grows in the deserts of the United States and Mexico.

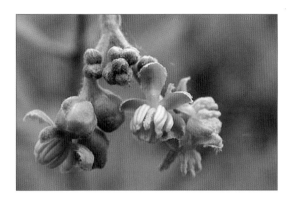

Native Americans and Aztecs used jojoba oil as an all-around healing substance for skin problems, eye infection, throat infection, and many other ailments. It has long been used for skin and hair care. Jojoba oil has a natural sun protection factor of UV4 and is quickly absorbed by the skin, leaving it smooth and soft. At the same time, because of its fatty acids, it protects and smoothes the skin, enhancing its elasticity and ability to retain moisture. It can be used for all skin types: dry, oily, and combination. This high-grade oil has a high level of vitamins E and F, minerals, and natural nourishment and care substances. It has become a secret weapon for repairing damaged hair.

Macadamia Nut Oil

The oil of the "queen of the nuts" has its origins in Hawaii, Australia, and the South Pacific and offers a wide range of restorative applications. Macadamia nut oil is suitable for all skin types and is considered a possible substitute for mink oil. What makes it unique is its very high level of palmidolein acid, usually found only in animal fat. Macadamia nut oil's similar constitution to the fatty acid of our skin makes it particularly

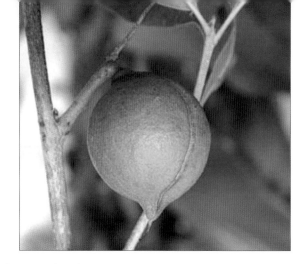

beneficial, leaving the skin more resistant to stress. It nourishes dry skin, softens calluses, activates the skin's metabolism, and helps the skin store moisture, leaving it silky and wonderfully soft. Because macadamia nut oil is absorbed slowly, it is an excellent massage oil.

Olive Oil

It doesn't take the most expensive body oil to satisfy the needs of skin and hair. High-grade, pure olive oil's fatty acid composition is similar to that of fatty tissue in the lower skin layers, and its natural vitamin E promotes elasticity and resilience. Warming the oil slightly increases its effectiveness. Olive oil is also used in naturopathy, as a base oil for the production of oil extracts such as St. John's wort oil, and as a massage and skin care oil. Adding olive oil to our skin cells strengthens cell membranes and leaves them less vulnerable to destruction by free radicals. In this way, olive oil is a natural antioxidant.

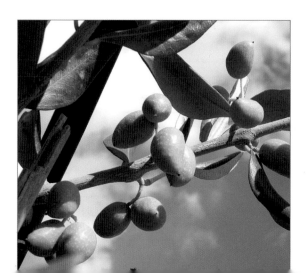

St. John's Wort Oil

St. John's wort oil is a maceration made from the petals of dotted St. John's wort, named for the black dots on the margins of its petals. A maceration is prepared by submersing a healing plant in oil and then leaving it in the sun until its active ingredients are transferred to the oil. St. John's wort has been known in Europe since the Dark Ages, when it was perceived to be a magic plant for preventing illness and misfortune. Doctors used the herb to treat wounds, muscle aches, bruises, frostbite, burns, and depression. Its calming, cleansing, antiseptic effect makes it well-suited for the treatment of dry, sensitive skin, especially for people who suffer from allergies. The oil also has a calming, rejuvenating effect on mood. On gray winter days, it brings a little sun and warmth to the skin. These characteristics make the oil useful for a wide range of stress treatments. Since St. John's wort has phototoxic characteristics, however, sun should be avoided following a massage using the oil.

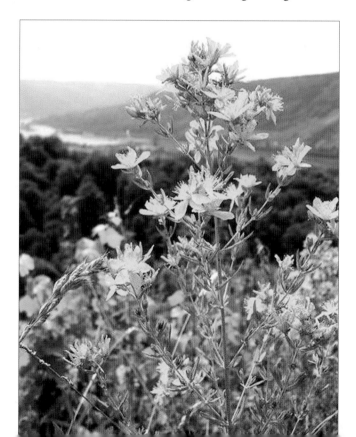

Evening Primrose Oil

The evening primrose gets its name from the fact that its petals open only in the evening, when it is pollinated by moths. Evening primrose oil is especially rich in unsaturated fatty acids, including about 10 percent gamma linolenic acid (GLA). GLA supports production of the body's metabolism regulators, thus supporting the skin's regenerative abilities. Cold-extracted evening primrose oil contains important amino acids, minerals, and vitamins, including vitamin E, a natural antioxidant. This revitalizing oil has overall positive effects on the functioning of the skin and is especially well suited for the treatment of skin allergies, eczema, and psoriasis. As an addition to massage oil, it is a relaxing and calming tonic for the nerves.

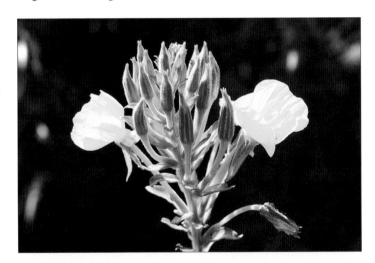

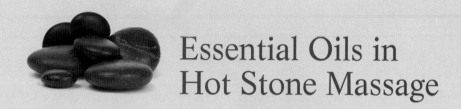

Essential Oils in
Hot Stone Massage

THE BASIC OILS LISTED in the previous chapter can also be enriched with essential oils for use in hot stone massage. When high-quality essential oils are combined with the basic oils, they have a heart-opening and calming effect on the psyche, as well as nurturing, regenerating, and vitalizing effects on the skin. In this way, body, soul, and spirit are equally affected.

Essential oils are highly concentrated plant extracts produced by distillation through steam, pressing, or extraction. Each plant's specific characteristics and qualities, many of which can be used as natural healing substances, are alive and concentrated in essential oils. Since each essential oil has its own particular scent and vibration, aromatherapy fulfills the desire for holistic therapy by addressing not only physical symptoms but also the spirit and soul of the person being massaged. Some essential oils are registered as natural healing substances, such as eucalyptus, peppermint, and pine. Rose, neroli, and lavender are equally well known for their superior balancing characteristics. The excellent restorative effects of essential oils have been recognized since the time of Cleopatra. Essential oils can disinfect the skin, stimulate the growth of cells and tissue, stop infections and mycoses of the skin, resolve

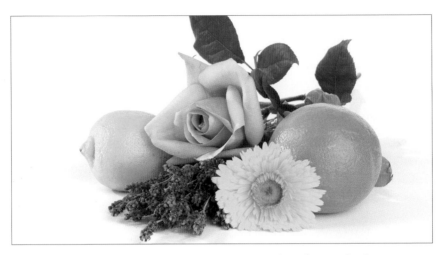

Essential oils hold the unique, healing quality of a specific plant.

lymph blockages, strengthen connective tissue, and stimulate the flow of energy in the body.

How Essential Oils Work

Essential oils have a very light molecular structure that enables them to penetrate deeply into the body's structure. From here they disperse themselves via blood circulation and are absorbed by the fluid in the lymph and cells, nerve pathways, and fatty and muscle tissue before being excreted via lungs and kidneys. Inhaled through the nose, essential oils reach the olfactory nerves, which translate their information into electrochemical signals that are transferred to the brain. The brain region, which controls emotional response to external influences, is closely linked to the production of hormones and the immune system, so essential oils are quickly distributed throughout the body and can thus affect the entire organism. In larger quantities, some essential oils have toxic effects, especially for the kidneys, liver, and central nervous system. For this reason, anyone wanting to work with essential oils should have basic knowledge of aroma science that includes what effect various oils have on the skin and psyche (whether they are calming or stimulating, balancing, or antisep-

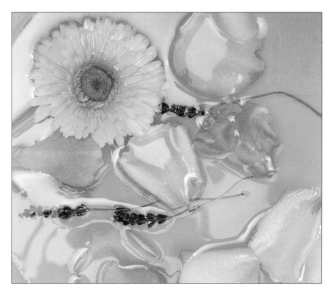

Essential oils are able to penetrate the deeper structures of the body.

tic) and how they interact with other essential oils. For example, lavender combined with bergamot and grapefruit is stimulating, but when used with neroli and rosewood it is more calming.

It is important to use high-quality oils. Label declarations tell a lot about the quality of the contents. Essential oils should be 100 percent pure and should, if possible, come from controlled organic cultivation or wild collection. Serious producers regularly subject their products to a rigorous series of tests. Misrepresentation of essential oils, especially in the higher price ranges such as rose oil, can be lucrative, so buyers need to be aware of the possibility that other essential oils or synthetic scents have been used. Significant price deviations should always be cause for questioning.

Essential oils should be stored in a cool, dark place in bottles made of brown or purple glass. Stored in this way, they will maintain their quality for about three years.

Here are some examples of essential oils well-suited for hot stone massage:

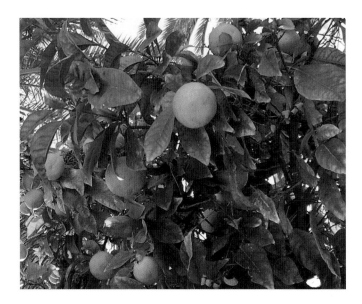

Orange (*Citrus sinensis*)

Oranges have one of the most popular aroma oils, with high therapeutic value. Orange oil contains significant amounts of vitamin C and carotene (vitamin A). Research has confirmed that orange oil stimulates the gland that produces the hormone melatonin, usually affected by light. The oil, derived from orange peels, contains the light-bringing, warming energy of the sun and brings light into dark moods. It soothes and nurtures the skin and is especially good for dry, irritated, or pollution-damaged skin. It stimulates lymph flow, resolves blockage in the tissue, and stimulates circulation. Moreover, it is very beneficial for older skin and for dry or calloused skin areas. Orange oil also has a calming effect on the stomach and intestines.

Rose (*Rosa damascena*)

The Damascene rose is cultivated primarily in France and Morocco. This robust rose resembles the hedge rose but is very mild and has the lowest toxicity of all oils. Rose essence is a prized—and pricey—beauty substance. To produce 2.2 pounds (1 kg) of pure rose oil

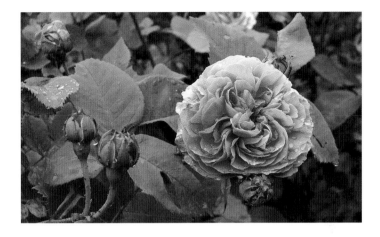

requires about 7,500 to 11,000 pounds (3,500 to 5,000 kg) of freshly flowering, handpicked rose petals.

Rose oil has a rejuvenating effect on skin and blood vessels, and encourages the growth of new tissue. It soothes the skin, alleviates redness and irritation, and stops infection. Rose oil cleanses, clears, heals, and is suitable for all skin types, especially infected, dry, or sensitive skin.

The *Rosa damascena* opens the heart for vibrations of love, humanity, and empathy. In crisis situations, for emotional depression, and in dealing with grief and death, rose is one of the most important substances of aromatherapy.

Lavender (*Lavandula angustifolia*)

The best areas for lavender cultivation are in the southern high plateaus of France, at an altitude between 2,500 and 4,000 feet (800 and 1,200 m). When buying lavender oil, be sure the label states "Real lavender (*Lavandula angustifolia*)." Otherwise you might end up buying *lavandin,* which is less suited for healing treatments and has a stimulating, rather than calming, effect. Lavender oil reduces infection, is antiseptic, and promotes regeneration of the skin. It encourages the formation of new skin cells and reduces the formation of scars. In natural beauty treatments, it is appreciated for its ability to balance the skin

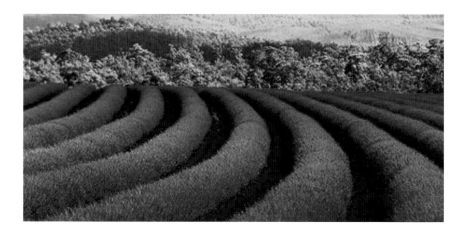

and stimulate circulation. It is suitable for all skin types, especially for dry skin. Its essence removes blockages in the skin by stimulating lymph flow. It promotes the formation of white blood cells, increases the body's natural defenses, and has an antiseptic effect on the breathing pathways. On the psychological level, lavender strengthens and calms the nerves, and helps to alleviate sleeping problems, anger, or nervousness.

Melissa (*Melissa officinalis*)

Melissa originally comes from the Mediterranean and the Orient, but it is common throughout Europe today. The oil has strong power to relieve

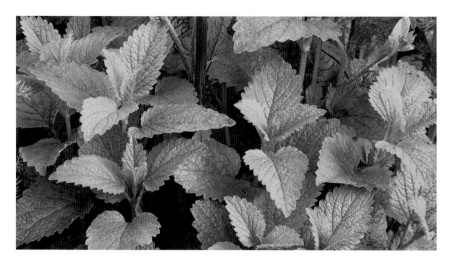

cramps and flatulence and is antiviral. It balances skin and hormones and prevents skin infection and allergies. Its calming effect on the nerves has been scientifically proved, and it is used to treat insomnia, stress, anger, and sadness. Melissa oil should not be used on pregnant women or for people who are undergoing homeopathic treatment.

Sandalwood (*Santalum album*)

Sandalwood is grown in eastern India, and its scent is popular with both men and women. Commercially, you will often find so-called West Indian sandalwood, or *Amyris* oil, which is significantly cheaper but much less effective. In its country of origin, sandalwood is an important healing substance of ayurveda, the traditional Indian medicine. It is very mild and alleviates dry, infected, itchy, or pollution-damaged skin. Sandalwood strengthens connective tissue, rejuvenates muscles, removes blockages in the lymph system, and stimulates the metabolism of the skin. Its scent is said to be an aphrodisiac, which is why it is often used in partner massage (together with jasmine and grapefruit). A massage with sandalwood oil is especially good for people who have difficulty with balance.

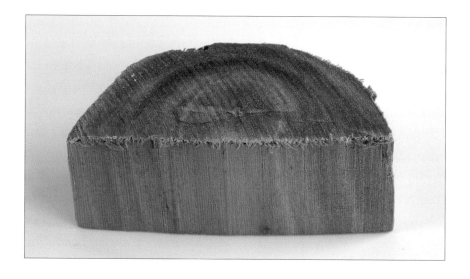

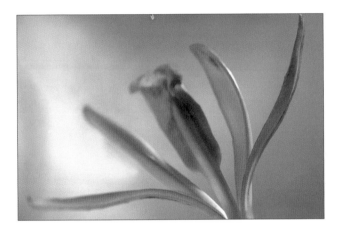

Vanilla (*Vanilla planifolia*)

Vanilla is a pod of a climbing orchid that originally comes from Latin America. When fresh, the vanilla pod has no scent; it is only the fermentation process that creates its dark color and sweet, balsamic scent. Vanilla provides energy, has rejuvenating and antiseptic effects, and stimulates digestion. Many people appreciate the calming effect of vanilla on spirit and soul, which is one reason why people reach for sweets containing vanilla in situations of anger or frustration.

Massage Oil Mixtures

For hot stone massage you can prepare a simple blend of either a basic oil (for example, sweet almond, jojoba, or macadamia nut oil) and an essential oil (for example, melissa or sandalwood), or add a combination of essential oils to the basic oil.

Essential scent notes are divided into head, heart, and base notes. Head notes are fresh, quickly disappearing scents. Typical of this category are orange and all citrus fragrances. Heart notes determine the theme of a scent mix. They are most often soft, intensive scents that "touch the heart." These include rose, lavender, or melissa. Base notes are those essences that can still be detected in the evening when they were applied in the morning. They are balsamic, earthy, and enduring scents, for example, sandalwood and vanilla. A good combination usually includes head, heart, and base notes.

Essential oils are added to the basic oils. To one-fourth cup (50 ml) basic oil, add at most 10 to 15 drops of essential oils. Although this ratio is generally suitable for the skin, it is always a good idea to first check for potential allergic reactions. Initially apply the oil to only a small area before spreading it over the entire body.

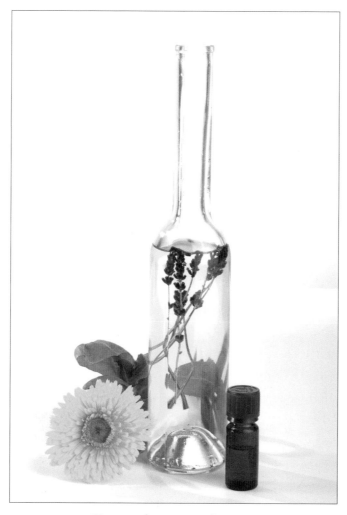

Homemade massage oil mixture

Sample Recipes for Mixtures with Essential Oils

¹/₄ cup (50 ml) base oil (for example, jojoba, sweet almond, or macadamia nut oil)

10–12 drops essential oil (for example, sandalwood, melissa, orange, or rose)

¹/₄ cup (50 ml) sweet almond oil

6 drops essential orange oil

5 drops essential lavender oil

4 drops essential sandalwood oil

¹/₄ cup (50 ml) jojoba oil

5 drops essential rose oil

3 drops essential lavender oil

3 drops essential orange oil

2 tablespoons (30 ml) jojoba oil

1¹/₄ tablespoons (20 ml) sweet almond oil

6 drops essential orange oil

5 drops essential rose oil

3 drops essential vanilla oil

One alternative to making these blends would be to purchase massage oil from specialized retailers. These should be 100 percent plant based, without synthetic scents, and without synthetic or chemically altered ingredients. There are a number of good oils that are well suited to hot stone massage, including Sensuality by Living Nature. This fragrant, calming, and balancing oil contains carrot, wheat germ, St. John's wort, marigold, lavender, and orange oils, as well as vitamin E. Or you may use gem massage oil Cairn Tara, an alchemical composition of high-grade, biologically based oils enriched with precious stones, herbal extracts, and essential oils. Seven different compositions of this type are available in specialized stores, including stimulating, sensitizing, or calming oils. (The Living Nature and Cairn Tara oils are pictured on page 52.)

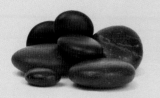 # Stone Warmer

TO WARM THE STONES, either add them to a large container (pot or bowl) filled with hot water, or use an electric stone heater with a thermostat. Warming the stones in a pot or bowl has the disadvantage that you will have to check the temperature using a thermometer and will need to keep refilling with hot water during the massage to maintain the stones at the desired temperature. Those who enjoy hot stone massage and want to use it on a regular basis should consider buying a warmer with a thermostat, which will maintain a constant water temperature. These heaters are available in specialty stores, and are not much different from electric meal warmers, or slow cookers, used in the food industry. The heater has two parts, the electrical part and the removable water reservoir. First fill the inset with water—the water will evenly distribute the heat. Then place the inset into the pot and cover it with a cloth to protect its coating. Place the stones on top of the cloth, completely immersed in water. Then choose the desired temperature on the thermostat. It will usually take about twenty minutes for stones to reach the desired temperature of 120 to 140°F (50 to 60°C).

After the massage, wipe out the machine with a wet cloth and wash the inset, if necessary, with disinfectant or dishwashing detergent.

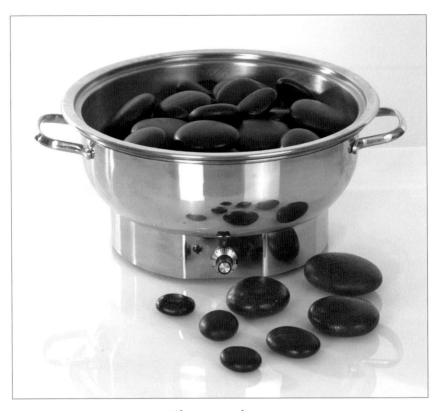

Electric stone heater

Massage oil should be kept in a glass bottle and is easiest warmed in a warmer for baby bottles. These machines also have a thermostat, allowing the oil to be kept at the desired temperature.

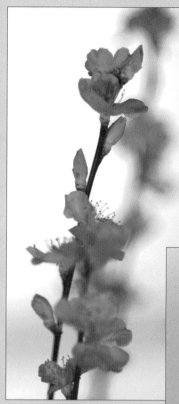

3
Preparing for
Hot Stone Massage

. . . .

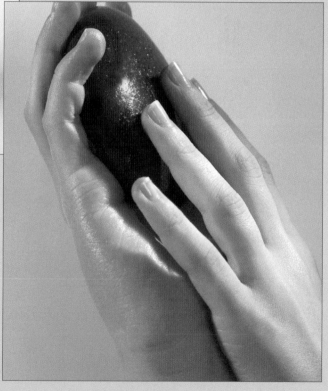

If a man is not patient in the small things,
his larger plans will be defeated.

Confucius

. . . .

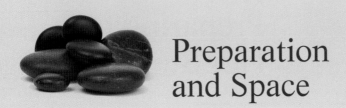

Preparation and Space

BEFORE YOU BEGIN THE MASSAGE, it is important to make a few preparations to ensure the treatment can be carried out calmly and harmoniously.

Atmosphere and Ambience

The room itself should be quiet, clean, well aired, and warm enough that the recipient of the massage can be relaxed and comfortable without clothing. Relaxation is important, indeed decisive, for all types of massage—the quieter and pleasanter the surroundings in which you work, the more effective will be your treatment. The lighting of the room should be dimmed, because bright lights make it impossible for the eyes to relax. If the recipient is lying on a massage table, it is important that the table be adjusted to your working height and accessible from all sides. If the massage is to be carried out on the floor or on a mattress, make sure there is enough room to sit on all sides.

Place the stones and the oil in a place you can reach without having to interrupt the massage for extended periods of time, and check before beginning the massage that the oil and stones are the right temperature. Have a blanket ready to cover the client, as well as a roll for

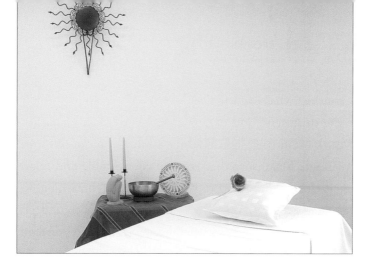

*Adding personal touches to the massage area creates
a welcoming space and enhances the treatment.*

the knees, or to support legs, head, or stomach. A massage table that
has been warmed with a warming bottle or blanket prior to the massage creates a comfortable atmosphere from the onset and is especially
pleasant for people who frequently feel cold.

Add your own atmosphere to the room: candles, flowers, gentle
relaxing music, a bowl of potpourri, or a few flower petals on the massage table—all radiate a welcoming feeling. Loving hands in nice surroundings create the rare and happy moments that make complete
relaxation possible.

State of Mind

You should be relaxed and feel good, ready to carry out the massage
with joy and care. The energy that you transfer through your hands is
weakened if you lack mental concentration. It is good to let your own
ego fade into the background during the massage, and to concentrate
fully on giving to the other. The quality of the touch and the effectiveness of the massage depend on your attitude, on the care and affection
you give to the recipient. When you concentrate fully, you will locate
sources of tension and energy imbalance more quickly. You will be able
to find the right touch for each body part and a rhythm that is ideal
for the recipient.

Also, consider what you will need for your own comfort. Allow enough time for the treatment, and organize things so you are able to work in peace. Wear loose-fitting, light clothing so that you can move freely during the massage. Make sure that you are comfortable and relaxed. Your well-being is closely connected to your posture and breathing. Keep your back straight, make your movements from the stomach and pelvis, and use the weight of your body to vary the depth of your movements. Let the stones work—because of their weight, you will need to apply only light pressure. Take deep and regular breaths, and enjoy the rhythm of the movements. A good massage demands complete concentration.

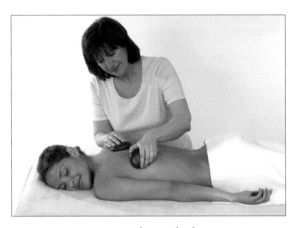

Your own comfort and relaxation
are important to giving a good massage.

Try to remain relaxed during the massage and concentrate on what you are doing. That way, you won't feel tense or tired after the massage.

Protection

Following a massage, therapists frequently experience symptoms that are similar to what their clients experienced beforehand. This can happen if you do not protect yourself sufficiently before and during the massage. In your protective measures you should include your internal and external attitude and posture, as well as energetic considerations. Especially in areas where there are energy blockages, you will find a density of energy. If you resolve these blockages in the recipient, you need to make sure you do not absorb these energies and burden yourself with them. You can create a protective barrier by making a conscious decision before the treatment that everything that belongs to the recipient will remain with that person, and everything that belongs to you will remain with you.

It also can be helpful to visualize yourself, your client, and the room surrounded by violet light. Violet is the color of cleansing and mental healing. In theosophic teaching, violet is the color of the "flame of transmutation" that burns all negative things and makes room for the new.

If you should become aware of foreign elements despite your precautions, reconnect with the recipient and essentially swap back energies. If the resolution of blockages releases energies that neither of you wants to claim, these still may be floating in the room. This may call for cleansing the room's energies through burning incense or sage or the sounding of singing bowls.

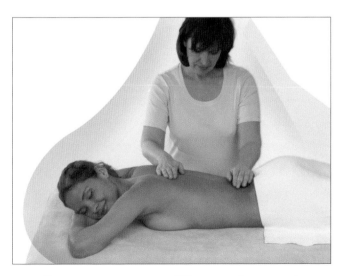

One way to protect yourself from negative energy is
to visualize a violet bubble that envelops your workspace.

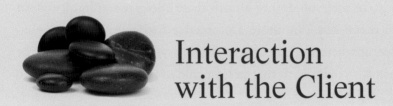

Interaction
with the Client

BEFORE THE MASSAGE it is useful to have a short conversation with the client, to allow him or her to fully "arrive." The willingness to completely enter into and enjoy a massage is reached by building trust. A friendly smile and conversation over a cup of tea sends the message that your client is in good hands.

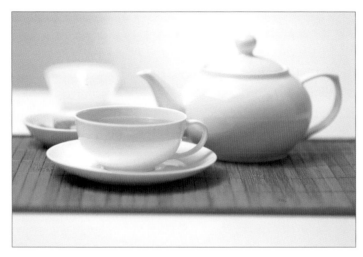

*Take a few moments before the massage to visit
with your client, perhaps over tea.*

Ask how the person is feeling, explain the sequence of the treatment, and ask whether there are any contraindications that might complicate the massage. Also ask about needs and preferences, and adjust the treatment accordingly. Before you use essential oils, be it in massage oil or as a scent in the room, first let the person smell the oil; even if the effectiveness spectrum is appropriate, if the recipient doesn't like the fragrance, it will have a negative influence on the entire massage. The same applies to your selection of music, since the same music that may cheer up one person can make another nervous or sad. Before you ask the recipient to lie down, offer the opportunity to use the bathroom.

After the massage, allow a bit of time for the person to continue to rest, while you remain within hearing distance. A cool towel on the face, soaked in water enriched with a drop of orange petal oil, can gently return the recipient to everyday life. A conversation and relevant observations conclude this wonderful treatment.

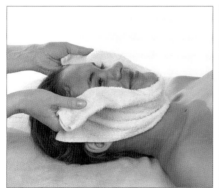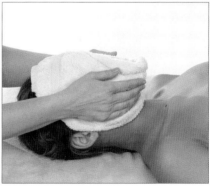

After the massage, you may want to place a towel soaked in cool water on the client's face.

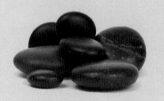

After the Massage

EVEN AFTER THE MASSAGE has come to an end, there are measures you can take to ensure that the client gets the most out of the massage and experiences a peaceful transition back to her day.

Resting

By allowing the recipient to rest for a while after the massage, the effectiveness of the massage is extended, and the recipient is not suddenly jarred from the state of relaxation. Quiet repose and relaxation change the blood pressure, which can lead to circulation problems when first returning to a vertical position. Getting up should be done slowly and carefully.

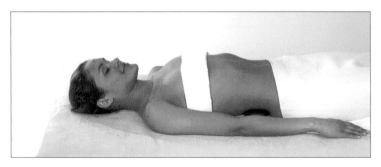

Allow the recipient ample time to rest
following the massage.

Fresh Air, Exercise, and Plenty of Liquids

Fresh air and movement help to stimulate circulation, and drinking water helps the body to transport and excrete toxins released by the massage. The best and most beneficial massage is not effective unless the body's transport system has enough fuel. If not, blockages and resettlement of the recently released toxins may result. When drinking, it is important to be sure that the water is pure, noncarbonated, and with a low mineral content. Pure water can draw and transport more toxins than water with high mineral content is able to process.

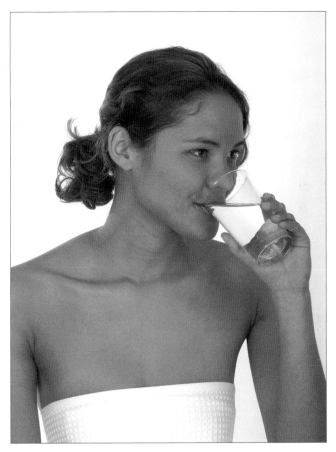

Drinking water helps the body eliminate toxins
released during massage.

Hot Stone Massage Preparation Checklist

CLIENT CARE

- Prepare a cup of tea, water, or juice
- Warm stones and oil and place them where they will be accessible
- Welcome the client
- Ask how the client is feeling
- Ask about illness
- Start file if necessary
- Inform recipient about the massage and sequence of treatment
- Ask about preference of essential oils
- Ask whether music or silence is preferred
- Cover body parts that are not being massaged
- Pay attention to the well-being of the client during the massage
- Refrain from conversation during the massage

MASSEUR/MASSEUSE ETIQUETTE

- Pay attention to cleanliness
- Have short nails (no nail polish)
- Maintain a fresh scent in the room (if necessary, use an aromatherapy burner or incense)
- Tie back long hair and remove jewelry from hands and wrists
- Be well rested and radiate calm

SPACE AND MATERIALS

- Warm, quiet, well-ventilated room
- Warm, dim light
- Comforting atmosphere in room
- Shower available, if possible
- Bottle warmer for heating oil
- Base and essential oils
- Warm blanket or warming bottle

• Towels, sheets, roll for the knees
• Warmer for basalt stones
• Eight stones 3 to 4 inches (9 cm) in diameter
• Twelve stones 2 to 3 inches (6 cm) in diameter
• Eight small, flat toe stones
• Tongs to remove the stones
• Gemstone massage stick (crystal wand)
• Chakra stones
• Preparations/supplies for cleansing the stones

AFTER THE MASSAGE

• Allow the client to rest for a few minutes, and keep him or her well covered
• Encourage client to drink plenty of water
• Recommend fresh air and movement

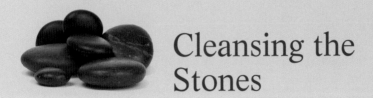

Cleansing the Stones

THE STONES USED IN THE MASSAGE absorb the energies of the client, and thus need to be cleansed carefully. As soon as the stones have cooled off, rinse them under cold running water to neutralize any accumulated charge. Never wash hot basalt, crystals, or gemstones in cold water; wait for them to cool completely. For a thorough cleaning you can then use a plant-based soap and add frankincense essential oil for disinfecting—10 drops oil to one-half cup (100 ml) soap. This technique, developed by Monika Grundmann, author of *Crystal Balance: A Step-by-Step Guide to Beauty and Health through Crystal Massage*, has proved very effective for the cleansing of massage stones. The basalt can also be boiled directly in the stone warmer. In the case of gems and crystals, however, we do not recommend this technique, as we have found that they often lose their strength as a result of this. For mechanical cleansing, the motto is: as much as possible, but as gently as possible.

You can then cleanse the basalt stones energetically by burning incense. The gems or crystals used in the chakra treatments can also be cleansed in resonant singing bowls and then allowed to rest on an amethyst or druze crystal (geode), where all stored information is deleted.

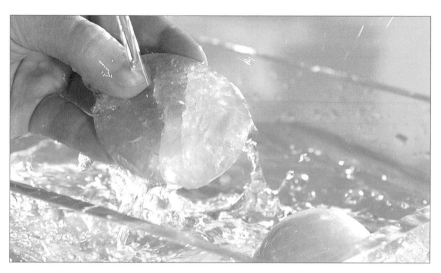

After the massage, rinse room-temperature stones under cold running water.

This ability of the amethyst to energetically cleanse other stones is one reason for the cleansing power of the color violet, mentioned earlier under the topic of protection. The other factor is finely dispersed iron in the quartz. The energy of these two parts (fiery iron and clearing quartz) intensely radiates throughout the many small crystal tips, then streams through the stone resting on top, and thus frees it of all that has adhered to it.

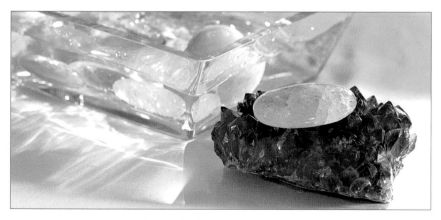

Energetic cleansing of the stones

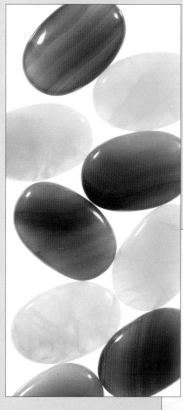

4
Hot Stone and
Gem Massage

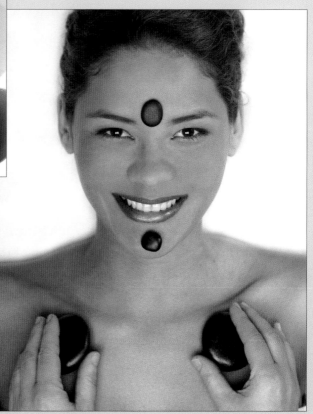

*When love and skill work together, expect
a masterpiece.*

John Ruskin

THE MASSAGES WE CARRY OUT WITH HOT STONES combine two decades of modern healing knowledge with traditional European, Chinese, Indian, and Native American teachings. However, this does not result, as one might at first assume, in a wild mixture of different cultures, since there is extensive overlap and parallels among the different methods. In the following pages we will describe a traditional Hawaiian hot stone massage.

The black basalt stones are warmed in water or a heater to a temperature of 120 to 140°F (50 to 60°C). At first the stones are placed on the body only to thoroughly warm it. Placing the stones on the energy centers of the hands, feet, forehead, neck, solar plexus, stomach, and abdomen causes the inherent powers of the stones to develop fully. This type of whole body massage is very intensive, since both the physical pressure of the stones and their energetic charge are felt immediately. The feeling of warm, oily stones on the skin is very pleasurable.

The massage itself follows this placing of the stones. Let the stones glide over the body as described in the following section, sometimes with a light and soft touch, sometimes with more pressure. All massage treatments should be given generously and slowly. Each individual stone, each individual movement should be clearly identifiable. To amplify the deep effect of the stones, you can knock or vibrate the stones during the massage to further release their warmth. This helps to gradually release blockages so that the body's energy can once again flow freely.

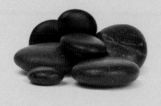

Body Massage— Lying on the Stomach

THE RECIPIENT IS LYING RELAXED, facedown, either on a massage table or on the floor. Stand or sit alongside and prepare the recipient for the massage. Then take the hot stones out of the water, dry them, and slide them under the body of the recipient. Slide three large and very flat stones under the middle of the body, approximately at the level of the chakras. With thin people, it is particularly important to make sure that the stones do not lie directly under bony body parts, since this can be very uncomfortable.

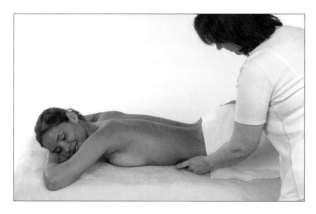

Placing stones under the body

Begin with the area of the root chakra. Once this stone is in place, continue with the area of the sacral chakra, then the solar plexus, and then the thymus chakra. In the thymus region we use two medium-size stones at the same level on the outside edges of the body. If you feel that you want to add or remove a few stones depending on the size of the stones and the recipient, then go ahead and follow your intuition.

A medium-size stone goes into each of the palms, and one each above the knee. If necessary, you can add a stone in each thigh area, as well as one to two stones in the shoulder-arm area or the neck, as well as a medium stone on the back of each knee and on the soles of the feet. If the client is comfortable, continue placing large stones on the back chakra areas, as well as on the thigh and calf, to achieve a complete warming.

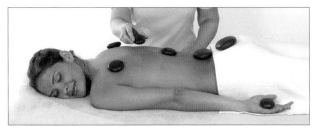

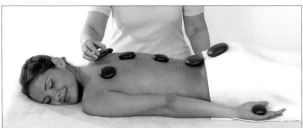

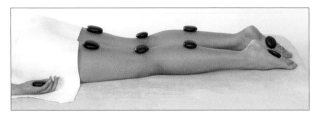

Placing the stones on the body

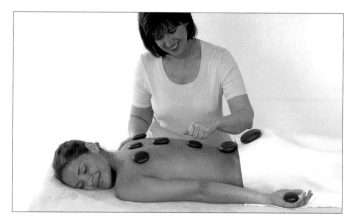

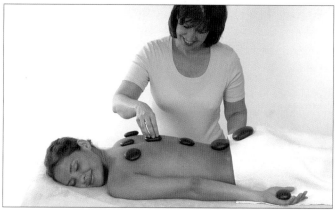

Knocking and vibrating the stones

Here, too, the deeper effects of the stones, as well as their warming effects, can be accelerated or amplified by lightly knocking on or vibrating the stones. Then allow the client to rest and warm up for a minute before beginning the massage.

To begin the massage, remove the stones from the back of the body, except for the stones in the palms and those on the soles of the feet. Now apply warm massage oil to back, legs, and arms. Take a large, warm stone and place it on the sacral area. This stone should be covered so that it can retain its warmth.

Back

Stand on the side of the massage table and place one hand on the sacral stone and the other between the shoulder blades. Now stimulate the sacral stone using light movement for about one minute, to make contact with the recipient. Then choose two medium stones, apply oil to them, and place them somewhere within easy reach. With the residual oil on your hands, massage in large strokes across the entire back. Then pick up the stones and stroke the entire length of the back using the stones. Then massage the sides and the ribs. Continue by rubbing the muscles around the shoulders using circular movements to create friction. Conclude by stroking the back, first with the stones and then with your hands.

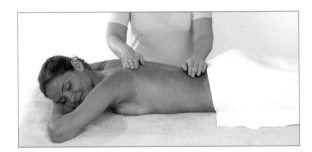

One hand between the shoulder blades and one vibrating a stone on the sacral area

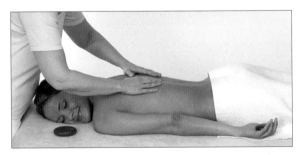

Stroking the back with hands

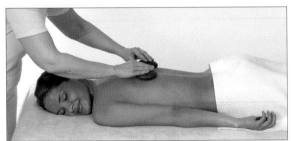

Stroking the back using hot stones

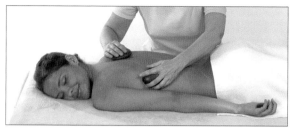

Massaging the sides

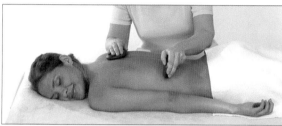

*Using downward strokes
in the gaps between the
ribs*

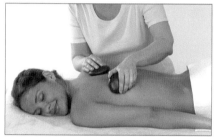 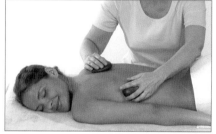

Massaging around the shoulder blades using circular movements (friction)

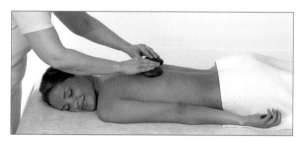

*Stroking the back using
hot stones*

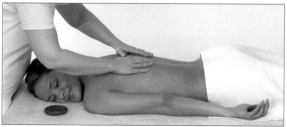

*Stroking the back with
hands*

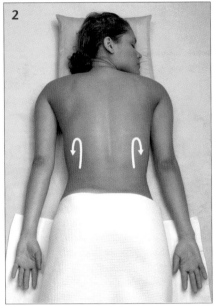

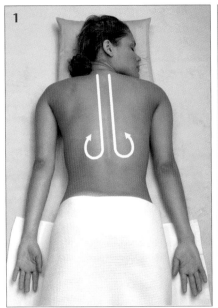

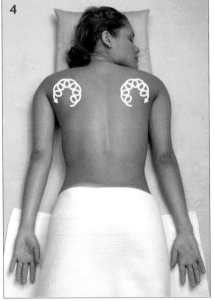

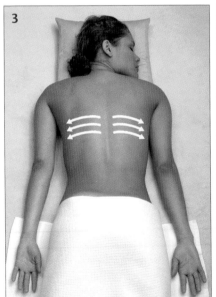

Overview of back massage

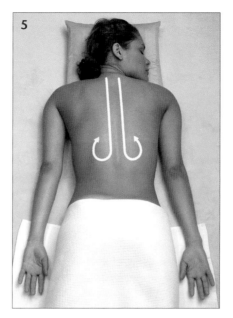

Conclusion of back massage

Arms

Choose two stones in a size that matches the diameter of the arms, apply oil to them, and place them within easy reach. Then use your hands to stroke one arm of the recipient. Now take the stones and use them to stroke the arm up to the shoulder and back. Follow this up with small circular movements, moving up from the wrist to the elbow, and from there back down to the wrist. Repeat this three times. From the elbow, continue in circling movements up along the upper arm, and then massage the shoulder area, again repeating this movement three times. Conclude by first stroking the arm with the stones, and then with your hands. Switch sides and massage the other arm in the same sequence.

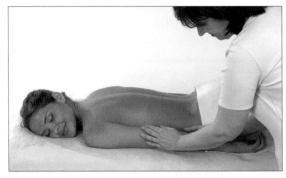

Stroking the arm with hands

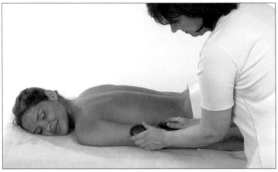

Stroking the arm using hot stones

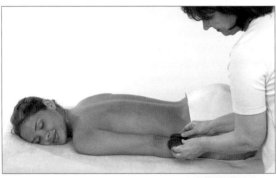

Small circles with hot stones

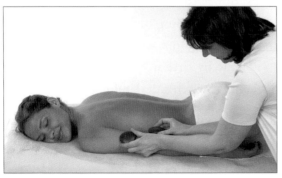

Stroking the arm using hot stones

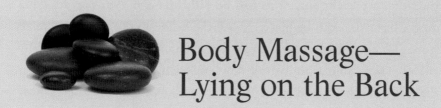

Body Massage—
Lying on the Back

BEFORE ASKING THE RECIPIENT TO TURN, remove all stones and place them back into the water. The recipient now turns over. Once the person is comfortable and relaxed, place the large basalt stones under the back, beginning with a large stone in the area of the sacral chakra, two large stones in the kidney area, and—as long as it feels comfortable—one in the area of the solar plexus. The next large stone is placed in the thymus area, although some people prefer two medium-size stones in this area.

Before proceeding with the massage, apply oil to the entire front of the body. Then place warm stones on the front of the body in the area of the chakras. The following sequence has proved effective: root, sacral,

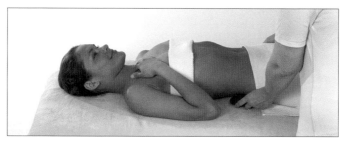

Placing hot stones under the body

solar plexus, as well as medium-size stones on the side liver and spleen chakras. Continue with heart, thymus, throat, nose, brow, and crown. The stone for the crown chakra does not have to be placed directly on the head, especially since this can be difficult with your partner lying down. Instead, it can be placed above the head, on the table. Use small stones for the throat chakra. Small, warm basalt stones are wonderfully effective for stimulating lymph flow, especially when placed between the individual toes, and stones behind the knees improve energy flow in the legs. Place small stones on the face near the sinuses and two freshly warmed stones in the hands.

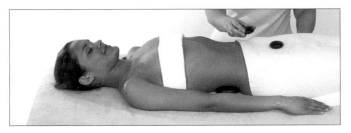

Placing chakra stones on the body

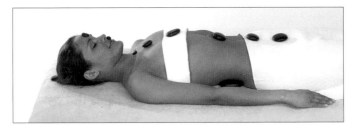

The chakra stones on the body

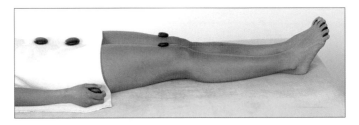

Hot stones on the knees and between the toes

Legs

Choose two stones of a suitable size, apply oil to them, and place them within easy reach. Begin stroking the leg from the ankle up, using your hands, before repeating the strokes with the stones. Then begin massaging the lower leg from the ankle, along the calf, up to the knee with gentle circling movements, and then return to the ankle. Repeat this three times, always making sure that the circles are oriented inward. Then massage to the left and right of the knee cap with circling movements and continue up to the thigh with gentle, circling movements that are oriented toward the inside. Make three paths—along the middle, the inside, and the outside—and repeat this three times. Conclude by using the stones in strokes that end at the ankle. Massage the ankle using the stone at a perpendicular angle, and then use the stone to massage the sole of the foot. Place the stone perpendicular and use small circles to massage first the front of the foot, before moving the stone along the length of the foot. Now put the stones aside and conclude the massage with hand strokes across the whole leg. Then switch sides and massage the other leg in the same sequence.

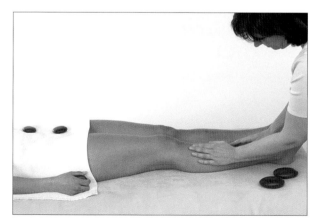

Stroking the leg with hands

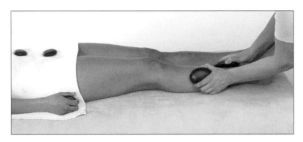

Stroking the leg using hot stones

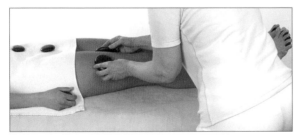

Circles toward the inside of the calf

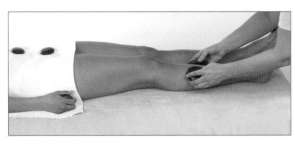

Circles on the sides of the knee

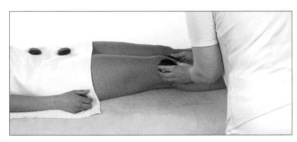

Circles toward the inside of the thigh

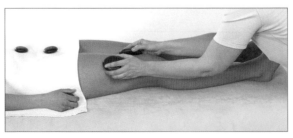

Stroking the leg using hot stones

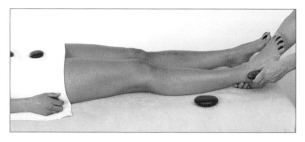

Massaging the ankle

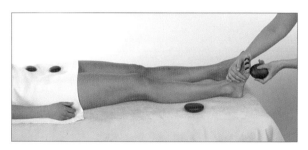

Massaging the sole of the foot

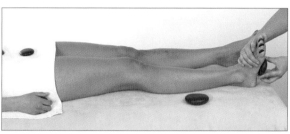

Massaging the bottom of the foot with small circles

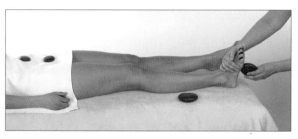

Pulling the stone down the length of the foot

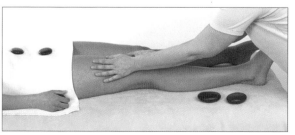

Stroking the leg with hands

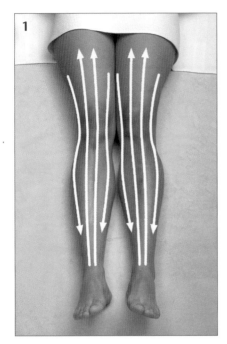

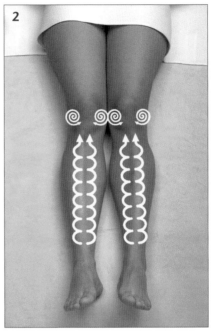

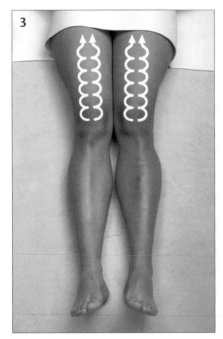

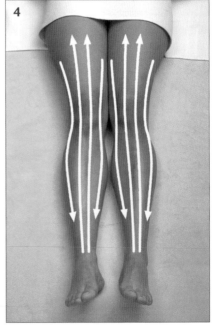

Overview of leg massage

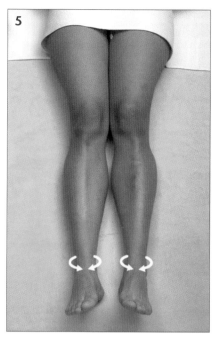

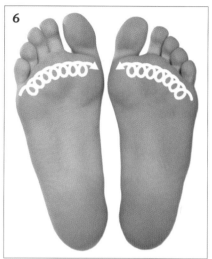

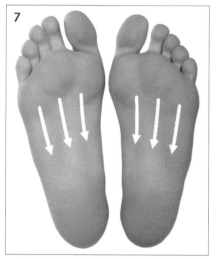

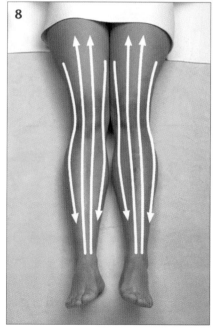

Arms

Choose two stones of an appropriate size, apply oil to them, and place them within easy reach. Begin by stroking the entire arm using your hands, making sure to include the shoulder area. Then repeat this process with the stones.

Now turn the arm so that the recipient's palm is facing upward, and stroke along the inside of the arm. Massage upward from the wrist with gentle circles, and conclude by stroking the stones along the arms to the wrist. Now put down one stone and use the other stone to massage the whole area of the palm. Then place the stone perpendicular and stroke the tendons in the palm, as well as the inside of the lower arm. Now put the stone aside and conclude with strokes along the whole arm using your hands. Then switch sides and massage the other arm in the same sequence.

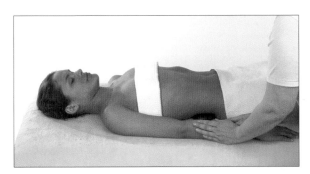

Stroking the arm with hands

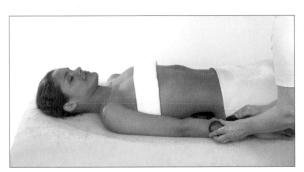

Stroking the arm using hot stones

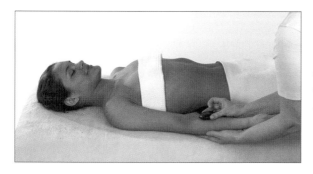

Stroking the inside of the arm using hot stones

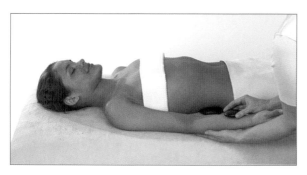

Massaging the inside of the arm in gentle circles

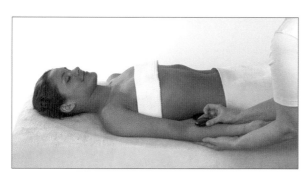

Stroking the inside of the arm using hot stones

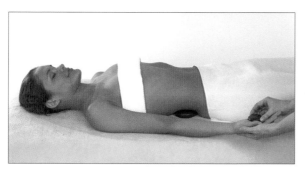

Massaging the palm

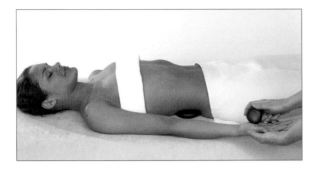

Stroking the palm

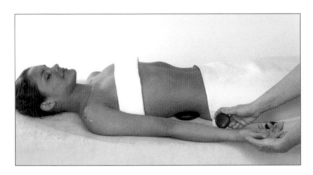

Stroking the tendons on the inside of the arm

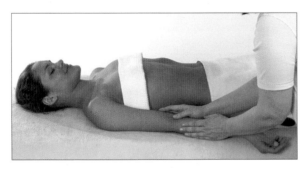

Stroking the arm with hands

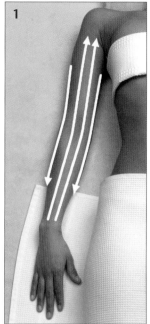

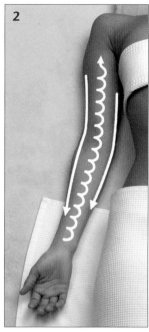

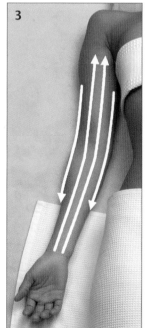

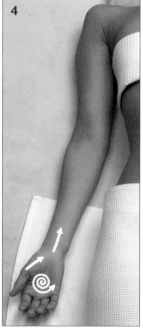

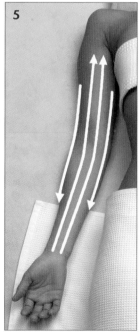

Overview of arm massage

Chest and Neck

Begin by removing the chakra stones from the brow and crown areas, because the head has to be turned slightly to the side for this part of the massage. Choose two stones for the chest and neck area, oil them, and put them within easy reach. Then stroke the upper chest using your hands before repeating the strokes with the stones. Now gently turn the

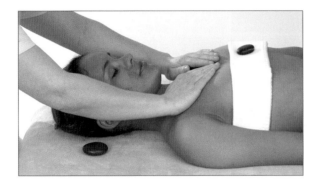

Stroking the chest with hands

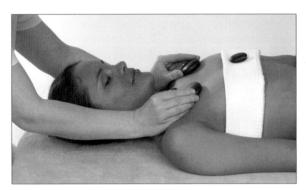

Stroking the chest using hot stones

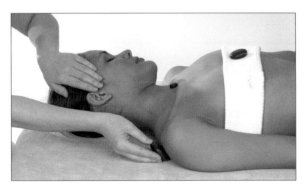

Circular massage from shoulder to neck

head to the side and massage each side in turn, keeping the second stone in the shoulder area of the resting side. Massage in circles from the shoulder to the neck. After that, place the stone perpendicular to the neck, pulling it along to the beginning of the trapezoid muscle, which is massaged with small circling movements. Conclude with strokes toward the shoulder, and massage the other side in the same way.

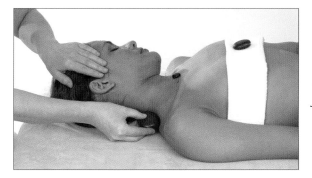

Pulling the stone up from shoulder to neck

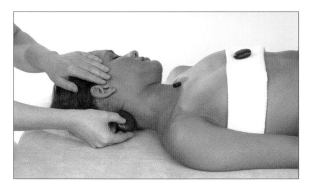

Circular massage at the beginning of the trapezoid

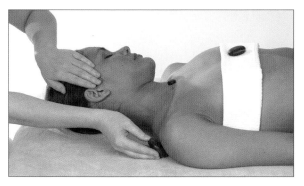

Stroking from neck to shoulder

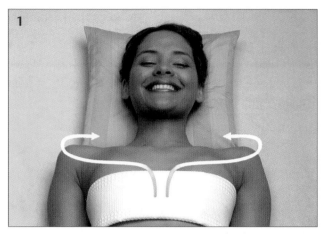

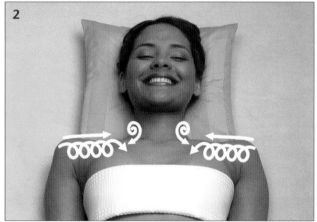

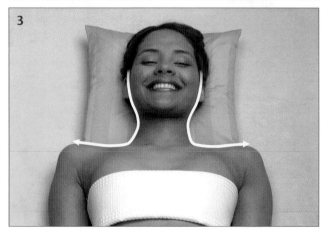

Overview of chest and neck massage

Head

Choose two stones about the size of the recipient's ear, and begin with circling movements on and behind the ear, using first your hands and then the stones. Then massage the ear with your hands. Use two fresh stones to massage the crown of the head in strokes and circling movements along the direction of the meridians.

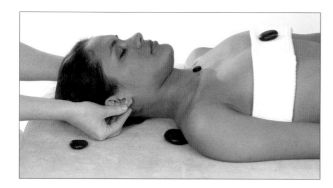

Circles on the ear with hands

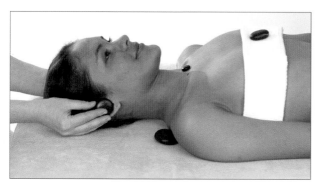

Circles on the ear using hot stones

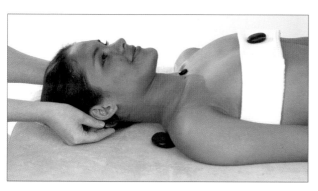

Circles behind the ear

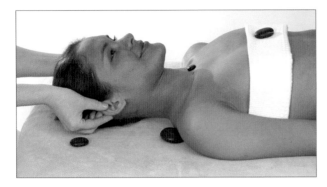

Massage on the ear using hands

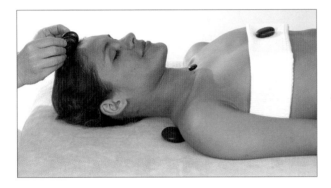

Stroking the head

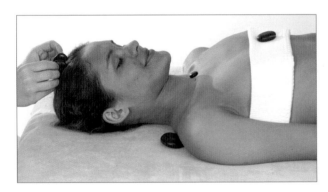

Massaging the head in circles

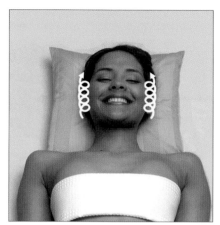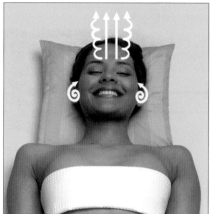

Overview of head massage

After finishing the massage of the head, conclude the whole body massage by applying light pressure to the shoulders, gently signifying completion of the body portion of the massage.

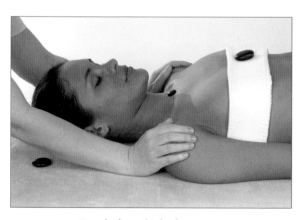

Concluding the body massage

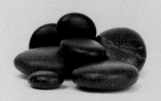 # Facial Massage

CHOOSE TWO SMALL, WARM BASALT STONES that are easy to hold in your fingers, or two warm gem sticks, or crystal wands. The gem sticks can be heated in the stone warmer up to 104°F (40°C). Before you begin this part of the massage, place small stones in the areas of the sinuses and the chakras.

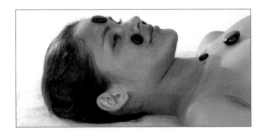

Then take the head of the recipient into your hands and allow it to rest there for a while.

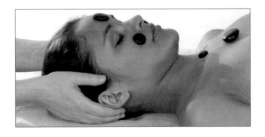

Use this time to focus completely on the person in front of you, and the massage ahead. Slowly and calmly take your hands away from the head, and then remove the stones from the face. Continue by applying a little oil to the face and gently stroking it from the center to the outer edge two or three times.

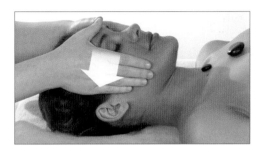

Now take the stones and begin stroking large, interconnected circles on the forehead.

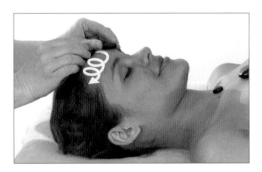

Then stroke the eyebrows from the center to the outer edge.

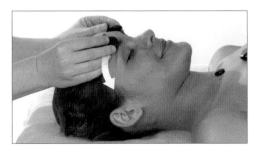

Stroke the frown lines from the root of the nose up along the forehead with alternating hands.

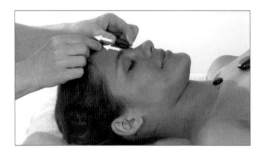

Now pull the stones along the temples and massage in small figure eights.

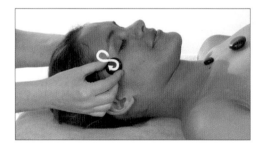

Now place the stones below the cheekbone and massage toward the ears in small circular movements. Continue with circular movements along the cheeks.

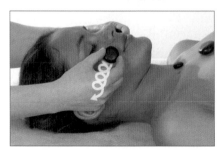
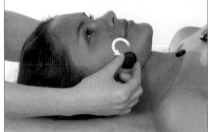

Then circle and stroke the area of the jaw from the middle of the face toward the outer edge.

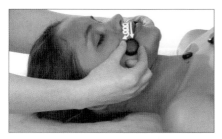 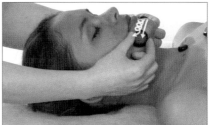

Put the stones aside and conclude the massage as you began it—with gentle strokes of your hands.

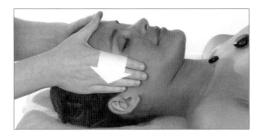

Then place the stones onto the face again and allow the recipient to rest for a little while.

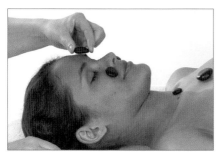 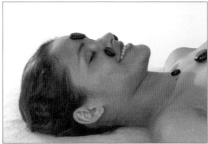

Of course you can follow your own intuition in this work, allowing knowledge from other massage areas to guide you, or simply play with the stones a bit.

Gemstone Massage Sticks

Gem sticks (or crystal wands) are cone-shaped gems, about 3 to 4 inches (8 to 10 cm) in length, and easy to hold. In addition to basalt, you can use the following stones for a facial massage.

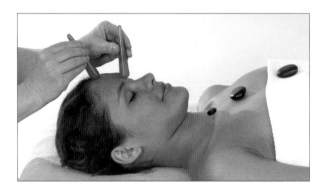

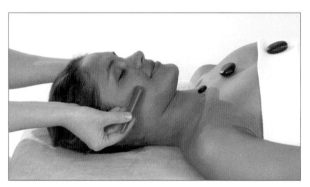

Facial massage with gem sticks

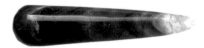

Amethyst helps with headaches, facial tension, and skin blemishes such as acne. Amethyst is considered a very good meditation stone, since it helps a free flow of thoughts and contributes to deep inner peace. Amethyst encourages both relaxation and a clear conscience.

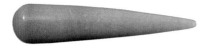

Aventurine cleanses connective tissue and skin, helps alleviate headaches caused by metabolism problems and irritated nerves, and helps to alleviate the effects of excess sun (both sunburn and sunstroke). Aventurine is one of the best stones for the entire head area and leaves the recipient with a glowing complexion. It also pushes obsessive thoughts out of the mind, thus helping to bring about deeper relaxation.

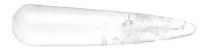

Rock crystal is well suited for balancing energies. Its positive influence on nerve pathways calms and relaxes places where there is an excess of energy, while acting as a stimulant in zones that lack energy—always in exactly the right amount. Rock crystal is very popular for facial massage because of its clearing characteristics. It is especially soothing to the eye area.

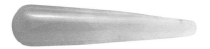

Rose quartz stimulates circulation in the skin. After a treatment with rose quartz the skin appears rosy and fresh and often feels velvety and smooth. Rose quartz strengthens our love for ourselves and helps us to accept ourselves as we are.

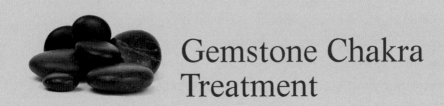

Gemstone Chakra Treatment

GEMSTONE CHAKRA TREATMENT IS USED at the end of many hot stone massages. The gems or crystals for this treatment are used at room temperature.

Sequence of the Treatment

Once again, stand or sit next to the client and focus on him. For this, it can be helpful to synchronize a few breaths with your client, which is a very simple way for people to enter into resonance with each other. Begin by using your left hand to connect with the root chakra. Recognize its energy and use your intuition to let your right hand select the correct stone from the bowl. Place this first stone on the pubic bone.

Next, feel the sacral chakra and again choose a stone based on your intuition, placing it about two finger widths below the navel. Place the stone for the solar plexus above the navel in the stomach area, and the one for the heart chakra in the middle of the body at the level of the heart. The thymus stone is placed in the upper third of the chest, precisely between the heart and the indentation of the larynx. Place the stone for the throat chakra just below the larynx

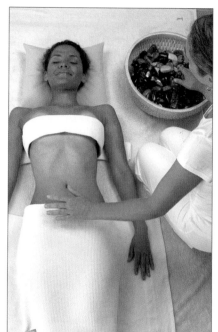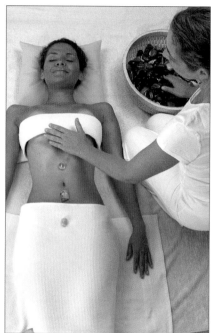

Intuitive choice of gemstones and crystals

into the little indentation, since it can be very unpleasant if placed directly on the larynx. The stone for the nose chakra is placed on the indentation of the upper lip. The stone for the brow chakra is placed between the eyebrows on the "third eye," while the stone for the crown chakra is placed above the head on the massage surface. Now allow the recipient to rest for a while with the stones in position.

To conclude the treatment, remove the chakra stones. Some may appear to be almost "stuck" to the recipient—allow those to rest a bit longer, since they are still working. Usually, when removing the last stone, the client will take a deep breath or open her eyes. Ask how she is feeling and encourage her to rest for a little while longer to enjoy the feeling. Also remember to exchange back any energies you might have accepted during the treatment and to cleanse the room and the stones.

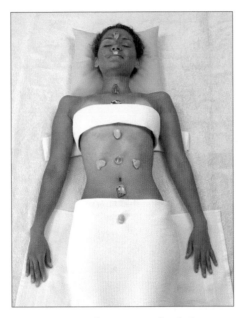

Resting with stones on the chakras

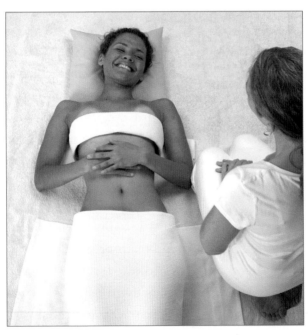

Concluding the treatment

Choosing the Gems

The gems and crystals described here are a small selection of stones that have proved effective in chakra treatment. It is not an exhaustive listing, so please feel free to add or reduce it as you find best.

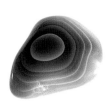

Agate is a classic protective stone. It helps to protect us against external influences and directs our attention within. It helps us to compose ourselves and to differentiate between significant and insignificant things. It also provides a feeling of safety. (*See also* Moss Agate.)

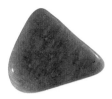

Amazonite balances mood swings and has a very harmonizing effect. It allows us to approach life with both intuition and vigilance. It helps us to act independently without always having to justify ourselves.

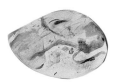

Amber transmits a worry-free, happy temperament and strengthens our confidence in ourselves. It helps us to like ourselves, spreads optimism, and supports us in allowing our inner light to shine.

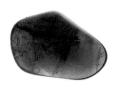

Amethyst is a popular meditation stone. It helps us to clear thoughts and feelings and to recognize internal and external realities, bringing us internal peace. Amethyst is also a valuable stone for dealing with grief.

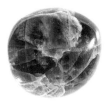

Apatite supports internal drive and thus increases motivation. It contributes to a secure and stable attitude, enabling us to be the "rock in the sea," a point from which we can encounter new things openly and alertly.

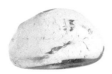

Aquamarine allows us to grow beyond ourselves. It allows us to see the world from a bird's eyes point of view, encouraging a long-term perspective. It helps us to keep an eye on ourselves and our goals.

Aventurine allows us to walk through life without being dragged down by worries. It is known as a stone that reduces stress; it builds a self-determined, worry-free existence. Because it frees the head of circular thoughts, it is also a good stone for falling asleep.

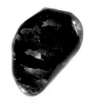

Bronzite is the stone for all who are experiencing stress, be they mothers or managers. It helps to create internal calm and, from that, the necessary energy and decisiveness to deal with stress in our everyday lives.

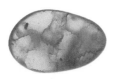

Orange-colored **calcite** strengthens self-confidence. Calcite helps whenever things are moving too slowly for us—it accelerates stalled developments and processes and helps us to accept change.

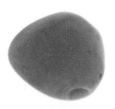

Carnelian motivates us to form our own opinions and to stand up for our views. It helps us to not let others put us down but to stand up to them. Carnelian also fosters our ability to process information.

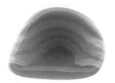

Chalcedony adds movement to our lives. It helps us design our lives with ease, happiness, and an open approach. It gives us the ability to reveal our internal selves.

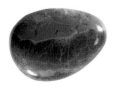

Chrysocolla helps us to recognize external influences and which ones negatively affect our balance. It helps us to distance ourselves from the problems of others and gives us the strength to stay true to ourselves and remain calm.

Chrysoprase helps build trust and gives a deep sense of comfort and belonging. It helps free us of negative influences. It is the right stone for an internal house cleaning, to sweep out things we have been wanting to release for a long time.

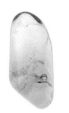

Citrine strengthens our joy of life and helps us to go beyond ourselves. It opens us up to new things and helps us to process our experiences. Citrine makes us aware of where the sweetness of life lies and gives us the strength to partake of it.

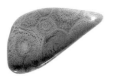

Fossilized **coral** assists personal expression and a strong ability to communicate, which foster a constructive approach to life. It supports a sense of community and the ability to listen to others.

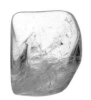

Danburite promotes a selfless love toward others but also helps us to accept ourselves as we are. It opens us for spiritual growth and allows us to discover our personal abilities.

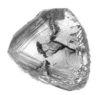

Diamond encourages a secure, strong approach to life. It increases our potential for mastering difficulties and for recognizing and resolving internal conflicts.

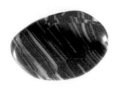

Dolomite helps us to remain grounded without becoming inflexible. It encourages agility of thought and the ability to translate thought into action in a quick and straightforward way. It supports us in doing what is necessary.

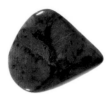

Dumortierite is also known as the "take it easy" stone. It helps us in difficult phases of our lives to take things a bit easier and to approach new challenges with confidence. It also helps us to have a relaxed interaction with whatever may come our way.

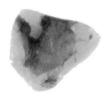

Emerald increases our artistic sensibility and our sensitivity to beauty. It helps us to make appropriate adjustments to life and to have a clear and open attitude. It shows us our goals in life and supports us when we have to overcome resistance to get there.

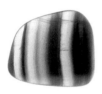

Fluorite helps us not to be influenced by external structures, and gives us the strength to free ourselves from confining life circumstances and patterns. It helps us to live in a free and decisive way and to be flexible in thought and deed.

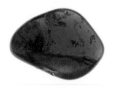

Garnet strengthens stamina and resistance, which helps us to master crises. It helps us not to lose ourselves, even when everything around us is collapsing. It brings energy and strength.

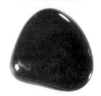

Heliotrope helps us to protect ourselves against mental attacks, to separate ourselves from negative influences, and to defend ourselves if necessary. In this way, it helps us to retain control over our lives.

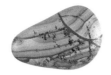

Landscape (or picture) jasper strengthens our stamina and our ability to deal with setbacks—by not giving up but returning to action with fresh energy.

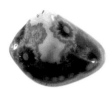

Ocean jasper assists recovery after severe stress. It supports better sleep, which helps us to deal with stress more effectively. Ocean jasper is beneficial for overall health—regulating bodily fluids and cell functions, strengthening the immune system, and promoting detoxification and excretion.

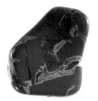

Red jasper strengthens our willpower and our ability to attain or achieve what we want out of life. It brings dynamism into our lives and makes us strong and courageous.

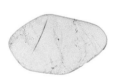

Kunzite helps us to give ourselves fully to obligations and challenges, as well as to pleasures. It helps us to empathize with others and be open to them. Kunzite is like a warm wave that we allow to carry us.

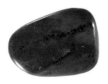

Lapis lazuli increases our ability to take responsibility for ourselves and for others. It helps us to be masters of our own domains and to be honest to others and to ourselves.

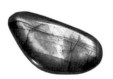

Labradorite stimulates the imagination and fosters creativity. It makes clear where it is worthwhile to exert energy and helps us to look at things realistically. It also helps us understand where we are in life—and why.

Magnesite helps us to relax and enjoy life, to channel the daily flood of thoughts and stop fretting. It erases bitterness and fosters the ability to smile at ourselves from time to time.

Malachite helps us to allow repressed emotions to rise slowly and gently so that we can process them well. It helps us to integrate desires and dreams into our lives.

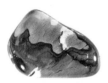

Mookaite brings a happy dynamic and decisiveness into life. It stimulates our internal wisdom and helps us to make use of it in our daily lives. It makes us want to realize long-held dreams.

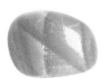

Moonstone strengthens intuitive abilities and improves fine perceptions. It helps us to feel deep, intensive feelings, and opens us to living these. It makes it possible to understand other points of view.

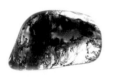

Moss agate is a stone of liberation, a shedding of structures and ties that have long since stopped serving us. It supports us in recognizing thoughts and resolutions that are outdated and letting them go, thus bringing new ideas and encouraging creativity.

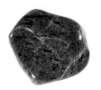

Nephrite creates balance and a peaceful internal posture. It makes us open to strangers and helps us to improve relationships by allowing our more balanced self to encounter our partner.

Obsidian encourages us to identify and process repressed memories. It loosens blockages and traumatic experiences and allows us to be more forgiving of our weak areas.

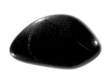

Onyx stimulates a healthy egotism and helps us to get our way. It stimulates a positive feeling of self-worth and helps us to differentiate useful from useless things. It helps us to change our perspective and define ourselves beyond our work.

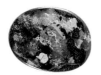

Opal brings the joy of living, and an optimistic, vital approach to life. It helps us to be able to enjoy the beautiful sides of life and makes us glad to be alive.

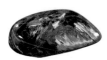

Pietersite helps us to navigate stormy times. It helps us to remain clearheaded in times of crisis and to be objective about difficult issues.

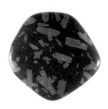

Porphyry increases our ability to reflect on ourselves and on our lives. It makes us more pensive and patient and encourages a calm and considered way of life. It gives us the ability to see ourselves as others see us.

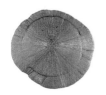

Pyrite helps us to recognize ourselves and the areas in which we would like to improve. It assists us in mastering conflict and supports a physical self-cleansing.

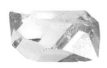

Rock crystal (clear quartz) is the stone of consciousness and clarity. It reveals the components of personality, thus helping each of us to approach our internal truth. It supports a pragmatic approach toward responsibilities.

Rose quartz amplifies sensitivity and warmth. It increases our ability to give love and attention where it is needed and to let things touch us in ways that allow us to grow and become stronger.

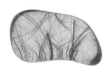

Rutilated quartz resolves tension in the chest that accompanies fear and worry. It frees us and allows us to breathe freely again.

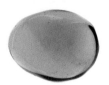

Smoky quartz is considered to be an antistress stone. It increases our ability to handle prolonged stress and helps resolve internal tensions. It gives us the ability to learn to value ourselves.

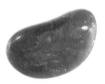

Rhodochrosite adds vivacity to our lives and helps us recognize and resolve avoidance strategies that cause illness. It allows us to take part in the lives of others and helps us to give ourselves and others a chance.

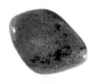

Rhodonite heals old and new wounds by allowing us to learn to forgive. It encourages problem solving and helps us to understand ourselves and others.

Ruby awakens passion. It is stimulating on all levels and lets us flower both inside and out. Ruby embodies "Life's longing for itself."

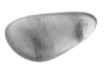

Serpentine protects us against outside influences. It helps us to set ourselves apart and break down internal tension, to find simple solutions to problems.

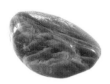

Sunstone helps us to say *yes* to life on all levels, especially to ourselves. It allows the sun to rise in our hearts and enables us to ignite a flame in the hearts of others.

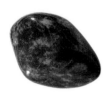

Thulite makes us adventurous and helps us to recognize and freely meet our needs. It gives us the ability to enjoy an endeavor and to dedicate ourselves heart and soul. It allows us to express our needs regardless of what others may think of them.

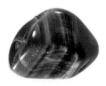

Tiger's eye helps us to keep a distance when necessary and to see things from a different perspective. This gives us a better overview in various situations.

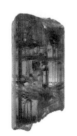

Tourmaline sets our life energy into motion. It protects us against external influences and helps us to integrate all aspects of our lives. Tourmaline brings a feeling of wholeness and helps us to accept ourselves.

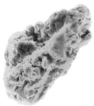

Turquoise conveys an understanding of the principle of cause and effect. It brings recognition of where in life we are our own cause and where we are being driven by other factors. Turquoise frees us from the role of victim and a belief in fate.

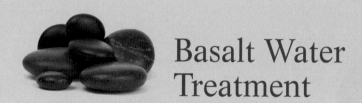

Basalt Water
Treatment

IN CONCLUSION, WE WOULD LIKE TO INTRODUCE you to one other way of using basalt stones, which originally was developed as the garnet water treatment. Because it is often difficult to find flat garnets that are suitable for this treatment, we began to use basalt. Basalt also stimulates the metabolism, and the warmed stones activate life energy (or chi) as much as garnet. For this treatment you will need about 25 to 30 small basalt stones.

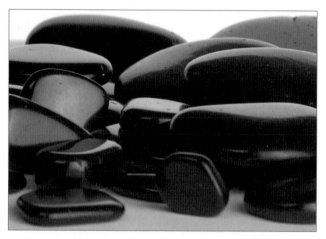

The flat shape of basalt stones lends itself well to this water treatment.

In the basalt water treatment the body is made slightly wet with lukewarm water all over. To do this, dip your hand in the water bowl and then stroke it gently over the body. Then watch where the water dries quickly, and where the body remains wet for a long time.

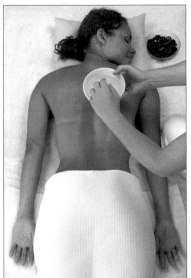
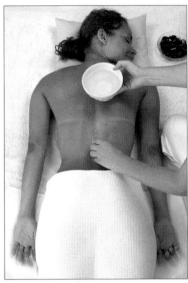
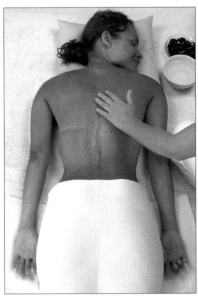

Applying water to the body

Body parts on which the water dries quickly are *high* energy zones—in contrast to areas that remain wet for a long period of time, which are *weak* energy zones.

To stimulate metabolism in the wet areas, place warm basalt stones precisely on those places, and leave them there for a while. In doing this, begin with the wettest parts. Sometimes you can observe even after the placing of just a few stones that all moist parts have begun drying more quickly.

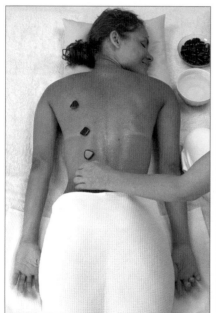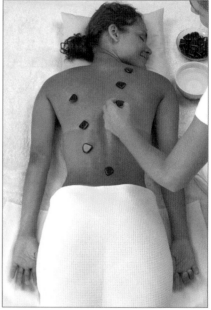

Placing warm basalt stones on the wet areas of the body

In this context, it is interesting to look at the wet body areas from a reflexology perspective. In doing so, it quickly becomes clear that these are not only energy-weak areas of our metabolism but that these body parts can indicate problems in very specific organs.

If the drying process takes a long time, don't hesitate to continue placing stones on the recipient until you have thoroughly covered all

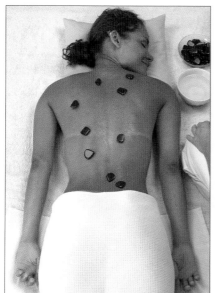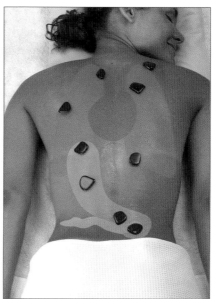

Using reflexology to gain greater insight into the weak-energy zones
of the body. Back reflexology zones: red = heart, violet = lungs,
beige = stomach, yellow = pancreas

wet spots. The stones should remain in place until the entire back is completely dry. Usually you will at that moment also have a reaction from your client (a deep breath, visible exhalation, content facial expression, a groan), showing you that you have achieved your goal. At this point you can remove the stones. Again, you may recognize the "stickiness" described in the chakra treatment above—some stones will seem to adhere slightly to the body. Allow these stones to rest on the body for a little while longer.

This treatment is very effective and produces surprisingly rapid results. People treated in this way feel very balanced and fit. Its effectiveness is confirmed by an anecdote in which one participant in a class did not feel well at all after this treatment, in contrast to all the other participants. At first we were at a loss as to how to explain this. After some discussion in the group, however, it turned out that

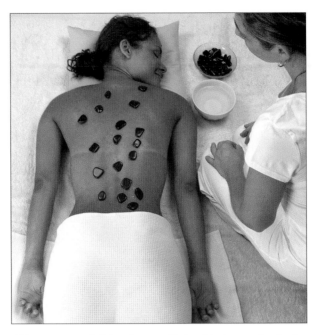

The stones are left in place until the skin is completely dry.

his partner had accidentally placed the stones on all the dry areas!

You should not apply basalt water treatment in the case of acute infection or of illness or problems accompanied by heat or swelling. This treatment can also be problematic for patients with hypertension or varicose veins (see contraindications of hot stone massage on page 16). If you are unsure, consult your client's doctor or healing practitioner.

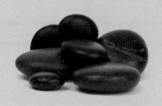

Conclusion

HOT STONE MASSAGE IS A FASCINATING COMBINATION of massage, energy treatment, and the beneficial effects of hot stones. The entire organism is recharged with energy and vitality, and the energy field is harmonized and strengthened. When combined with the scent of essential oils, or complemented by the use of crystals and gemstones,

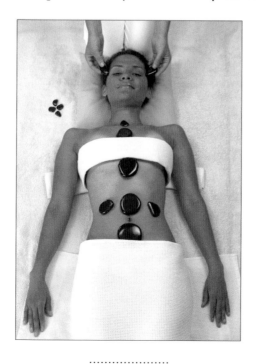

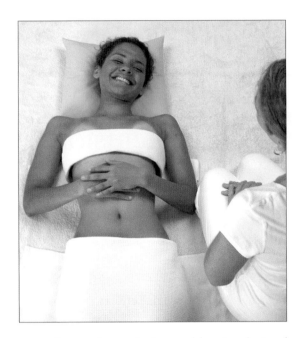

this combination of intensive and pleasurable stimulation leads to comprehensive relaxation of all senses, and a deep, holistic experience.

Don't be confused as to which is the correct, the original, or the most authentic of all ancient hot stone massages. Many providers claim to be offering the "original." But the fact is that all massage techniques that contribute to the well-being of a person are valid. Ideas often arise simultaneously in the morphic field, in a "hundredth monkey" way, especially if the time for them is ripe. In massage, the same maxim as in medicine applies: "He who heals is correct."

We hope that with this book we have been able to build bridges. Bridges between simple massage techniques and the art of massage. Bridges between modern perspectives and ancient teachings.

As you massage, be attentive and open, allowing your intuition to be your guide. Simply following massage instructions will not be enough to create an unspoken connection with your client. Massage can be a mindless series of actions or a meditative experience. Trust yourself.

And now give your creativity free rein. Try it out.

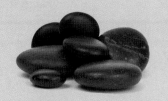

Acknowledgments

MANY HELPING HANDS ARE NECESSARY TO MAKE this kind of book a reality. To this end, we would like to thank most sincerely all those who worked on this book and were always there when needed. Although we cannot list all of you by name, you know who you are—and you can be sure we thank you with all our hearts!

A very special thanks goes to our families for their support and understanding. We especially thank Dirk Jochum for his steady help and successful photography research; Dorothea Sokpolie, our hand model, for her helpful collaboration and precision during the photo shoots; as well as our model, Tiana Cristina Souza de Oliveira, for her endless patience during long photo sessions, where even the hot stones occasionally got chilled.

A special thanks also goes to Ines Blersch for her kind and loving way with all of us, and her ability to always get Cristina to smile her beautiful smile. This book lives as a result of Ines Blersch's professional vision through the camera and her creative artistic design. We also thank Petra Ucakar for makeup and Ulrike von Gemmingen for her support in the photo studio. Thanks also to Eva Maria Lohner for her review of the first manuscript and for helpful conversations.

We also thank Fred Hageneder for the excellent graphics and

Andreas Lentz of Neue Erde, who published the German edition of this book.

Despite all this, this book would not have come about had Michael Gienger not given us the inspiration for it. To him go our biggest thanks as friend, teacher, and companion, and of course as first-rate editor, photo editor, and publisher.

Illustration Credits

Photographs by Ines Blersch with the following exceptions:

Arco Digital Images: 11, 22 (top, second from left), 62 (bottom), 63
www.digitalstock.de: 44 (top), 55, 62 (top)
Dragon Design, GB: 19, 22 (bottom), 30, 31 (editing), 34
GEOPHOT, Bernhard Edmaier: 46
Historical sources: 4, 8, 26, 27
Annette Höggemeier, Botanical Garden, Ruhr University, Bochum:
      53, 54 (top)
www.imagepoint.biz: 48
Dirk Jochum: 71, 143
Ute Keil: 43 (bottom)
Immo Lang: 60
Annette Partz: 49
www.pixelio.de: viii, 6, 7, 21, 22 (top, first and third from left), 28, 52
      (bottom), 54 (bottom), 56, 61
The artist/creator of the illustration on page 31, appearing in many
      other books and Internet sites, unfortunately could not be identi-
      fied. The addition of the correspondence to the human body was
      done by Dragon Design.

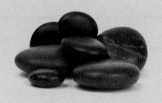

About the Authors

Dagmar Fleck

Dagmar Fleck, born in 1967, is the mother of two children, a crystal/gem consultant, head of the Cairn Elen Life Schools in Schwaebisch Alb, and owner of the mineral wholesale shop Laurin's Garden. She began her work in the field of natural healing and therapy early on and was founding principal of a school for healing practitioners. She has completed training in homeopathy, transpersonal psychology, foot reflexology, individual therapy, and communication. She became fascinated by crystals and their applications in the 1990s during a lecture

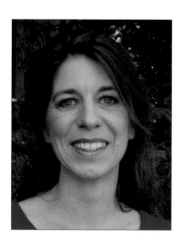

by Michael Gienger, the founder of analytic crystal healing. Convinced by his scientifically founded presentation on the effectiveness of gems, she became one of the first students to complete his two-year course in crystal healing, after which she spent four years as his teaching assistant. Dagmar is a founding member of the Crystal Healing Society in Germany (1995) and in 1997 founded, together with Michael Gienger, Petra Endres, Franca Bauer, and Annette Jakobi, the Cairn Elen Life Schools. Aside from gem and crystal healing courses, the Cairn Elen Life Schools aim to connect ancient natural healing knowledge with modern discoveries. Dagmar is also a cofounder of the Cairn Elen Network (1998), a free network of therapists and consultants. In 2005, Dagmar, together with Franca Bauer, took over the organization of the Cairn Elen Life Schools. Today she leads seminars and courses in gem/ crystal healing and related areas and is involved in the fair trade of minerals. She has worked for many years to create a quality seal for correctly labeled stones.

Contact:

Dagmar Fleck
Rossgumpenstr. 10, 72336 Balingen-Zillhausen, Germany
Telephone: (49) 7435 919932
Fax: (49) 7435 919931
dagmar@cairn-elen.de
www.laurinsgarten.de

Liane Jochum

Liane Jochum, born in 1959, is the mother of three children and director of ACADEMIA balance, which offers specialized training in natural spa treatments, ayurveda, and wellness in Buseck bei Giessen, Germany. Until the mid-1990s she worked as a journalist in natural healing and medicine. During this time she was responsible for the content of informational broadcasts on these subjects, as a freelance

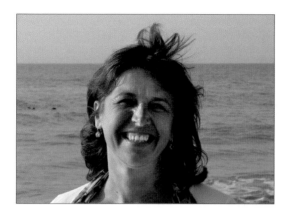

journalist for a number of television broadcasters. Aside from natural healing Liane has always been a proponent of natural beauty treatments and a holistic approach to wellness, which ultimately led to her current position. After conventional training in spa therapies, she studied natural healing preparations, herbs, and makeup. She was certified as a natural cosmetic wellness and spa therapist, as well as an ayurveda wellness therapist, and earned a number of massage certifications: hot stone massage, gemstone massage, singing bowl massage, and Asian steam-heated herb pouch massage. In early 2000 Liane fulfilled her dream of founding her own institute—the ACADEMIA balance, a technical college for natural spa treatments, ayurveda, and wellness. Today, she is happy to share her knowledge in trainings and seminars. She lectures at international events and is a contributing author for a number of trade publications.

Contact:

Liane Jochum
Grasweg 27, 35418 Buseck
Telephone: (49) 6408 5003 99
Fax: (49) 6408 5003 80
info@academia-balance.de
www.academia-balance.de

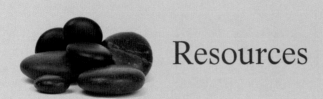

Resources

Basalt Stones, Stone Heaters, and Chakra Gem Sets

Hot Stone Hut
207-1425 Marine Drive
West Vancouver, BC V7T 1B9
Canada
503-420-9819
info@hotstonehut.com
www.hotstonehut.com

River Rock Massage
3097 62nd Street
Shellsburg, Iowa 52332
319-364-7748
riverrockmassage@fmtcs.com
www.riverrockmassage.com

Rub Rocks
5069 David Strickland Rd
STE #103
Fort Worth, Texas 76119
817-483-9860
John@rubrocks.com
www.rubrocks.com

**Turley International Resources
(TIR) Massage Stone Division**
4322 South 80th Street
Mesa, Arizona 85212
866-553-0596 • 480-516-4736
info2@tirmassagestone.com
www.tirmassagestone.com

Gems and Crystals

Heaven and Earth, LLC
P.O. Box 249
East Montpelier, VT 05651
800-942-9423 • 802-476-4775
heavenandearth@earthlink.net
www.heavenandearthjewelry.com

Starborn Creations
2550 West Highway 89A, Suite 8
Sedona, Arizona 86336
800-749-5498 • 928-204-2400
sales@starborncreations.com
www.starborncreations.com

Massage Oils

Aubrey Organics
4419 N. Manhattan Avenue
Tampa, Florida 33614
800-282-7394
www.aubrey-organics.com

Living Nature
P.O. Box 193
Kerikeri
Northland
New Zealand
64 (0) 9 407 7895
www.livingnature.com

Cairn Tara
Andrea Stanton
205 North Plain Road
Great Barrington, MA 01230
413-297-2802

Recommended Reading

Gienger, Michael. *Crystal Massage for Health and Healing.* Findhorn, Scotland: Findhorn Press, 2006.

———. *Crystal Power, Crystal Healing: The Complete Handbook.* New York: Sterling, 1998.

———. *Healing Crystals: The A–Z Guide to 430 Gemstones.* Findhorn, Scotland: Findhorn Press, 2005.

Welch, Ricky. *Aurum Manus: The "Golden Hands" Method of Crystal-based Holistic Massage.* Findhorn, Scotland: Findhorn Press, 2006.

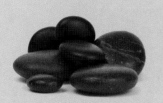

Index